MedicalCenter.com

I0407486

The Key Facts
On Cancer Prevention

The Key Facts on Cancer: Volume IV

Everything You Need to Know About Cancer Prevention

-Usable Medical Information for the Patient-

By Patrick W. Nee

www.MedicalCenter.com

Published by:

MedicalCenter.com

96 Walter Street/ Suite 200

Boston, MA 02131, USA

Tel: 617-354-7722

www.MedicalCenter.com

manager@medicalcenter.com

The Key Facts on Cancer Series

Table of Contents

Chapter 1: Introduction

What is Cancer?

Cancer is a term used for diseases in which abnormal cells divide without control and are able to invade other tissues. Cancer cells can spread to other parts of the body through the blood and lymph systems.

Cancer is not just one disease but many diseases. There are more than 100 different types of cancer. Most cancers are named for the organ or type of cell in which they start - for example, cancer that begins in the colon is called colon cancer; cancer that begins in melanocytes of the skin is called melanoma.

Cancer types can be grouped into broader categories. The main categories of cancer include:

- **Carcinoma**- cancer that begins in the skin or in tissues that line or cover internal organs. There are a number of subtypes of carcinoma, including adenocarcinoma, basal cell carcinoma,squamous cell carcinoma, and transitional cell carcinoma.

- **Sarcoma** - cancer that begins in bone, cartilage, fat, muscle, blood vessels, or other connective or supportive tissue.

- *Leukemia* - cancer that starts in blood-forming tissue such as the bone marrow and causes large numbers of abnormal blood cells to be produced and enter the blood.
- *Lymphoma and myeloma* - cancers that begin in the cells of the immune system.
- *Central nervous system cancers* - cancers that begin in the tissues of the brain and spinal cord.

<u>Origins of Cancer</u>

All cancers begin in cells, the body's basic unit of life. To understand cancer, it's helpful to know what happens when normal cells become cancer cells.

The body is made up of many types of cells. These cells grow and divide in a controlled way to produce more cells as they are needed to keep the body healthy. When cells become old or damaged, they die and are replaced with new cells. However, sometimes this orderly process goes wrong. The genetic material (DNA) of a cell can become damaged or changed, producing mutations that affect normal cell growth and division. When this happens, cells do not die when they should and new cells form when the body does not need them. The extra cells may form a mass of tissue called a tumor.

Not all tumors are cancerous; tumors can be benign or malignant.

- ***Benign tumors*** aren't cancerous. They can often be removed, and, in most cases, they do not come back. Cells in benign tumors do not spread to other parts of the body.

- ***Malignant tumors*** are cancerous. Cells in these tumors can invade nearby tissues and spread to other parts of the body. The spread of cancer from one part of the body to another is called metastasis.

Some cancers do not form tumors. For example, leukemia is a cancer of the bone marrow and blood.

Cancer Statistics

A report from the nation's leading cancer organizations shows that rates of death in the United States from all cancers for men and women continued to fall between 2005 and 2009, the most recent reporting period available.

Estimated new cases and deaths from cancer in the United States in 2013:

- *New cases*: 1,660,290 (does not include nonmelanoma skin cancers)
- *Deaths*: 580,350

The risk of developing many types of cancer can be reduced by practicing healthy lifestyle habits, such as eating a healthy diet, getting regular exercise, and not smoking. Also, the sooner a cancer is found and treatment begins, the better the chances are that the treatment will be successful.

Chapter 2: Cancer Vaccines

- Cancer vaccines are designed to boost the body's natural ability to protect itself, through the immune system, from dangers posed by damaged or abnormal cells such as cancer cells.

- The U.S. Food and Drug Administration (FDA) has approved two types of vaccines to prevent cancer: vaccines against the hepatitis B virus, which can cause liver cancer, and vaccines against human papillomavirus types 16 and 18, which are responsible for about 70 percent of cervical cancer cases.

- The FDA has approved one cancer treatment vaccine for certain men with metastatic prostate cancer.

- Researchers are developing treatment vaccines against many types of cancer and testing them in clinical trials.

What are vaccines?

Vaccines are medicines that boost the immune system's natural ability to protect the body against "foreign invaders," mainly infectious agents, that may cause disease.

The immune system is a complex network of organs, tissues, and specialized cells that act collectively to defend the body. When an infectious microbe invades the body, the immune system recognizes it as foreign, destroys it, and "remembers" it to prevent another infection should the microbe invade the body again in the future. Vaccines take advantage of this response.

Traditional vaccines usually contain harmless versions of microbes—killed or weakened microbes, or parts of microbes—that do not cause disease but are able to stimulate an immune response against the microbes. When the immune system encounters these substances through vaccination, it responds to them, eliminates them from the body, and develops a memory of them. This vaccine-induced memory enables the immune system to act quickly to protect the body if it becomes infected by the same microbes in the future. The immune system's role in defending against disease-causing microbes has long been recognized. Scientists have also discovered that the immune system can protect the body against threats posed by certain damaged, diseased, or abnormal cells, including cancer cells.

How do vaccines stimulate the immune system?

White blood cells, or leukocytes, play the main role in immune responses. These cells carry out the many tasks required to protect the body against disease-causing microbes and abnormal cells.

Some types of leukocytes patrol the circulation, seeking foreign invaders and diseased, damaged, or dead cells. These white blood cells provide a general—or nonspecific—level of immune protection.

Other types of leukocytes, known as lymphocytes, provide targeted protection against specific threats, whether from a specific microbe or a diseased or abnormal cell. The most important groups of lymphocytes responsible for carrying out immune responses against such threats are B cells and cytotoxic (cell-killing) T cells.

B cells make antibodies, which are large secreted proteins that bind to, inactivate, and help destroy foreign invaders or abnormal cells. Most preventive vaccines, including those aimed at hepatitis B virus (HBV) and human papillomavirus (HPV), stimulate the production of antibodies that bind to specific, targeted microbes and block their ability to cause infection. Cytotoxic T cells, which are also known as killer T cells, kill infected or abnormal cells by releasing toxic chemicals or by prompting the cells to self-destruct (a process known as apoptosis).

Other types of lymphocytes and leukocytes play supporting roles to ensure that B cells and killer T cells do their jobs effectively. These supporting cells include helper T cells and dendritic cells, which help activate killer T cells and enable them to recognize specific threats.

Cancer treatment vaccines are designed to work by activating B cells and killer T cells and directing them to recognize and act against specific types of cancer. They do this by introducing one or more molecules known as antigens into the body, usually by injection. An antigen is a substance that stimulates a specific immune response. An antigen can be a protein or another type of molecule found on the surface of or inside a cell.

Microbes are recognized by the immune system as a potential threat that should be destroyed because they carry foreign or "non-self" antigens. In contrast, normal cells in the body have antigens that identify them as "self." Self antigens tell the immune system that normal cells are not a threat and should be ignored.

Cancer cells can carry both self antigens and cancer-associated antigens. The cancer-associated antigens mark the cancer cells as abnormal, or foreign, and can cause B cells and killer T cells to mount an attack against them.

Cancer cells may also make much larger amounts of certain self antigens than normal cells. Because of their high abundance, these self antigens may be viewed by the immune system as being foreign and, therefore, may trigger an immune response against the cancer cells.

What are cancer vaccines?

Cancer vaccines are medicines that belong to a class of substances known as biological response modifiers. Biological response modifiers work by stimulating or restoring the immune system's ability to fight infections and disease. There are two broad types of cancer vaccines:

- Preventive (or prophylactic) vaccines, which are intended to prevent cancer from developing in healthy people; and
- Treatment (or therapeutic) vaccines, which are intended to treat an existing cancer by strengthening the body's natural defenses against the cancer.

Two types of cancer preventive vaccines are available in the United States, and one cancer treatment vaccine has recently become available.

How do cancer preventive vaccines work?

Cancer preventive vaccines target infectious agents that cause or contribute to the development of cancer. They are similar to traditional vaccines, which help prevent infectious diseases, such as measles or polio, by protecting the body against infection. Both cancer preventive vaccines and traditional vaccines are based on antigens that are carried by infectious agents and that are relatively easy for the immune system to recognize as foreign.

What cancer preventive vaccines are approved in the United States?

The U.S. Food and Drug Administration (FDA) has approved two vaccines, Gardasil® and Cervarix®, that protect against infection by the two types of HPV—types 16 and 18—that cause approximately 70 percent of all cases of cervical cancer worldwide. At least 17 other types of HPV are responsible for the remaining 30 percent of cervical cancer cases. HPV types 16 and/or 18 also cause some vaginal, vulvar, anal, penile, and oropharyngeal cancers.

In addition, Gardasil protects against infection by two additional HPV types, 6 and 11, which are responsible for about 90 percent of all cases of genital warts in males and females but do not cause cervical cancer.

Gardasil, manufactured by Merck & Company, is based on HPV antigens that are proteins. These proteins are used in the laboratory to make four different types of "virus-like particles," or VLPs, that correspond to HPV types 6, 11, 16, and 18. The four types of VLPs are then combined to make the vaccine. Because Gardasil targets four HPV types, it is called a quadrivalent vaccine. In contrast with traditional vaccines, which are often composed of weakened whole microbes, VLPs are not infectious. However, the VLPs in Gardasil are still able to stimulate the production of antibodies against HPV types 6, 11, 16, and 18.

Cervarix, manufactured by GlaxoSmithKline, is a bivalent vaccine. It is composed of VLPs made with proteins from HPV types 16 and 18. In addition, there is some initial evidence that Cervarix provides partial protection against a few additional HPV types that can cause cancer. However, more studies will be needed to understand the magnitude and impact of this effect.

Gardasil is approved for use in females to prevent cervical cancer and some vulvar and vaginal cancers caused by HPV types 16 and 18, and for use in males and females to prevent anal cancer and precancerous anal lesions caused by these HPV types. Gardasil is also approved for use in males and females to prevent genital warts caused by HPV types 6 and

11. The vaccine is approved for these uses in females and males ages 9 to 26. Cervarix is approved for use in females ages 9 to 25 to prevent cervical cancer caused by HPV types 16 and 18.

The FDA has also approved a cancer preventive vaccine that protects against HBV infection. Chronic HBV infection can lead to liver cancer. The original HBV vaccine was approved in 1981, making it the first cancer preventive vaccine to be successfully developed and marketed. Today, most children in the United States are vaccinated against HBV shortly after birth.

Have other microbes been associated with cancer?

Many scientists believe that microbes cause or contribute to between 15 percent and 25 percent of all cancers diagnosed worldwide each year, with the percentage being lower in developed than developing countries.

The International Agency for Research on Cancer (IARC) has classified several microbes as carcinogenic (causing or contributing to the development of cancer in people), including HPV and HBV. These infectious agents—bacteria, viruses, and parasites—and the cancer types with which they are most strongly associated are listed in the table below.

Infectious Agents	Type of Organism	Associated Cancers
Hepatitis B virus (HBV)	Virus	Hepatocellular carcinoma (a type of liver cancer)
Hepatitis C virus (HCV)	Virus	Hepatocellular carcinoma (a type of liver cancer)
Human papillomavirus (HPV) types 16 and 18, as well as other HPV types	Virus	Cervical cancer; vaginal cancer; vulvar cancer; oropharyngeal cancer (cancers of the base of the tongue, tonsils, or upper throat); anal cancer; penile cancer; squamous cell carcinoma of the skin
Epstein-Barr virus	Virus	Burkitt lymphoma; non-Hodgkin lymphoma; Hodgkin lymphoma; nasopharyngeal carcinoma (cancer of the upper part of the throat behind the nose)

Kaposi sarcoma-associated herpesvirus (KSHV), also known as human herpesvirus 8 (HHV8)	Virus	Kaposi sarcoma
Human T-cell lymphotropic virus type 1 (HTLV1)	Virus	Adult T-cell leukemia/lymphoma
Helicobacter Pylori	Bacterium	Stomach cancer; mucosa-associated lymphoid tissue (MALT) lymphoma
Schistosomes (*Schistosoma hematobium)*	Parasite	Bladder cancer
Liver flukes (*Opisthorchis viverrini)*	Parasite	Cholagniocarcinoma (a type of liver cancer)

How are cancer treatment vaccines designed to work?

Cancer treatment vaccines are designed to treat cancers that have already developed. They are intended to delay or stop cancer cell growth; to cause tumor shrinkage; to prevent cancer from coming back; or to eliminate cancer cells that have not been killed by other forms of treatment.

Developing effective cancer treatment vaccines requires a detailed understanding of how immune system cells and cancer cells interact. The immune system often does not "see" cancer cells as dangerous or foreign, as it generally does with microbes. Therefore, the immune system does not mount a strong attack against the cancer cells.

Several factors may make it difficult for the immune system to target growing cancers for destruction. Most important, cancer cells carry normal self antigens in addition to specific cancer-associated antigens. Furthermore, cancer cells sometimes undergo genetic changes that may lead to the loss of cancer-associated antigens. Finally, cancer cells can produce chemical messages that suppress anticancer immune responses by killer T cells. As a result, even when the immune system recognizes a growing cancer as a threat, the cancer may still escape a strong attack by the immune system.

Producing effective treatment vaccines has proven much more difficult and challenging than developing cancer preventive vaccines. To be effective, cancer treatment vaccines must achieve two goals. First, like traditional vaccines and cancer preventive vaccines, cancer treatment vaccines must stimulate specific immune responses against the correct target. Second, the immune responses must be powerful enough to overcome the barriers that cancer cells use to protect themselves from attack by B cells and killer T cells. Recent advances in understanding how cancer cells escape recognition and attack by the immune system are now giving researchers the knowledge required to design cancer treatment vaccines that can accomplish both goals.

Has the FDA approved any cancer treatment vaccines?

In April 2010, the FDA approved the first cancer treatment vaccine. This vaccine, sipuleucel-T (Provenge®, manufactured by Dendreon), is approved for use in some men with metastatic prostate cancer. It is designed to stimulate an immune response to prostatic acid phosphatase (PAP), an antigen that is found on most prostate cancer cells. In a clinical trial, sipuleucel-T increased the survival of men with a certain type of metastatic prostate cancer by about 4 months.

Unlike some other cancer treatment vaccines under development, sipuleucel-T is customized to each patient. The vaccine is created by isolating immune system cells called antigen-presenting cells (APCs) from a patient's blood through a procedure called leukapheresis. The APCs are sent to Dendreon, where they are cultured with a protein called PAP-GM-CSF. This protein consists of PAP linked to another protein called granulocyte-macrophage colony-stimulating factor (GM-CSF). The latter protein stimulates the immune system and enhances antigen presentation. APC cells cultured with PAP-GM-CSF constitute the active component of sipuleucel-T. Each patient's cells are returned to the patient's treating physician and infused into the patient. Patients receive three treatments, usually 2 weeks apart, with each round of treatment requiring the same manufacturing process. Although the precise mechanism of action of sipuleucel-T is not known, it appears that the APCs that have taken up PAP-GM-CSF stimulate T cells of the immune system to kill tumor cells that express PAP.

How are cancer vaccines made?

All cancer preventive vaccines approved by the FDA to date have been made using antigens from microbes that cause or contribute to the development of cancer. These include antigens from HBV and specific types of HPV. These antigens are proteins that help make up the outer surface of the viruses. Because only part of these microbes is used, the resulting vaccines are not infectious and, therefore, cannot cause disease.

Researchers are also creating synthetic versions of antigens in the laboratory for use in cancer preventive vaccines. In doing this, they often modify the chemical structure of the antigens to stimulate immune responses that are stronger than those caused by the original antigens.

Similarly, cancer treatment vaccines are made using antigens from cancer cells or modified versions of them. Antigens that have been used thus far include proteins, carbohydrates (sugars), glycoproteins or glycopeptides (carbohydrate-protein combinations), and gangliosides (carbohydrate-lipid combinations).

Cancer treatment vaccines are also being developed using weakened or killed cancer cells that carry a specific cancer-associated antigen or immune cells that are modified to express such an antigen. These cells can come from a patient himself or herself (called an autologous vaccine, such as sipuleucel-T) or from another patient (called an allogeneic vaccine).

Other types of cancer treatment vaccines are made using molecules of deoxyribonucleic acid (DNA) or ribonucleic acid (RNA) that contain the genetic instructions for cancer-associated antigens. The DNA or RNA can be injected alone into a patient as a "naked nucleic acid" vaccine, or researchers can insert the DNA or RNA into a harmless virus. After the naked nucleic acid or virus is injected into the body, the DNA or RNA is taken up by cells, which begin to manufacture the tumor-associated antigens. Researchers hope that the cells will make enough of the tumor-associated antigens to stimulate a strong immune response.

Scientists have identified a large number of cancer-associated antigens, several of which are now being used to make experimental cancer treatment vaccines. Some of these antigens are found on or in many or most types of cancer cells. Others are unique to specific cancer types.

Do cancer vaccines have side effects?

Vaccines intended to prevent or treat cancer appear to have safety profiles comparable to those of traditional vaccines. However, the side effects of cancer vaccines can vary among vaccine formulations and from one person to another.

The most commonly reported side effect of cancer vaccines is inflammation at the site of injection, including redness, pain, swelling, warming of the skin, itchiness, and occasionally a rash.

People sometimes experience flu-like symptoms after receiving a cancer vaccine, including fever, chills, weakness, dizziness, nausea or vomiting, muscle ache, fatigue, headache, and occasional breathing difficulties. Blood pressure may also be affected.

Other, more serious health problems have been reported in smaller numbers of people after receiving a cancer vaccine. These problems may or may not have been caused by the vaccine. The reported problems have included asthma, appendicitis, pelvic inflammatory disease, and certain autoimmune diseases, including arthritis and systemic lupus erythematosus.

Vaccines, like any other medication affecting the immune system, can cause adverse effects that may prove life threatening. For example, severe hypersensitivity (allergic) reactions to specific vaccine ingredients have occurred following vaccination. However, such severe reactions are quite rare.

Can cancer treatment vaccines be combined with other types of cancer therapy?

Yes. In many of the clinical trials of cancer treatment vaccines that are now under way, vaccines are being given with other forms of cancer therapy. Therapies that have been combined with cancer treatment vaccines include surgery, chemotherapy, radiation therapy, and some forms of targeted therapy, including therapies that are intended to boost immune system responses against cancer.

Several studies have suggested that cancer treatment vaccines may be most effective when given in combination with other forms of cancer therapy. In addition, in some clinical trials, cancer treatment vaccines have appeared to increase the effectiveness of other cancer therapies.

Additional evidence suggests that surgical removal of large tumors may enhance the effectiveness of cancer treatment vaccines. In patients with extensive disease, the immune system may be overwhelmed by the cancer. Surgical removal of the tumor may make it easier for the body to develop an effective immune response.

Researchers are also designing clinical trials to answer questions such as whether a specific cancer treatment vaccine works best when it is administered before chemotherapy, after chemotherapy, or at the same time as chemotherapy. Answers to such questions may not only provide information about how best to use a specific cancer treatment vaccine but also reveal additional basic principles to guide the future development of combination therapies involving vaccines.

What additional research is under way?

Although researchers have identified many cancer-associated antigens, these molecules vary widely in their capacity to stimulate a strong anticancer immune response. Two major areas of research aimed at developing better cancer treatment vaccines involve the identification of novel cancer-associated antigens that may prove more effective in stimulating immune responses than the already known antigens and the development of methods to enhance the ability of cancer-associated antigens to stimulate the immune system. Research is also under way to determine how to combine multiple antigens within a single cancer treatment vaccine to produce optimal anticancer immune responses.

Perhaps the most promising avenue of cancer vaccine research is aimed at better understanding the basic biology underlying how immune system cells and cancer cells interact. New technologies are being created as part of this effort. For example, a new type of imaging technology allows researchers to observe killer T cells and cancer cells interacting inside the body.

Researchers are also trying to identify the mechanisms by which cancer cells evade or suppress anticancer immune responses. A better understanding of how cancer cells manipulate the immune system could lead to the development of new drugs that block those processes and thereby improve the effectiveness of cancer treatment vaccines. For example, some cancer cells produce chemical signals that attract white blood cells known as regulatory T cells, or Tregs, to a tumor site. Tregs often release cytokines that suppress the activity of nearby killer T cells. The combination of a cancer treatment vaccine with a drug that would block the negative effects of one or more of these suppressive cytokines on killer T cells might improve the vaccine's effectiveness in generating potent killer T cell antitumor responses.

Chapter 3: Human Papillomavirus (HPV) Vaccines

- Human papillomaviruses (HPVs) are a group of more than 150 related viruses, certain types of which can cause cancer.
- The Food and Drug Administration-approved vaccines Gardasil® and Cervarix® are highly effective in preventing infection with certain types of HPV.
- HPV vaccination has the potential to reduce cervical cancer deaths around the world by as much as two-thirds, and to prevent anal cancer in males and females. Gardasil can also prevent genital warts.

What are human papillomaviruses?

Human papillomaviruses (HPVs) are a group of more than 150 related viruses. They are called papillomaviruses because certain types may cause warts, or papillomas, which are benign (noncancerous) growths. Some types of HPV are associated with certain types of cancer. These are called "high-risk," oncogenic, or carcinogenic HPVs.

Of the more than 150 types of HPV, more than 40 types can be passed from one person to another through sexual contact. Transmission can occur in the genitals, anal, or oral regions. Although HPVs are usually transmitted sexually, doctors cannot say for certain when infection occurred. About 6 million new genital HPV infections occur each year in the United States. Most HPV infections occur without any symptoms and go away without any treatment over the course of a few years. However, HPV infections sometimes persist for many years, with or without causing detectable cell abnormalities.

What kinds of cancer are related to HPV infection?

Infection with high-risk HPV is the major cause of cervical cancer. Almost all women will have an HPV infection at some point, but very few will develop cervical cancer. The immune system of most women will usually suppress or eliminate HPVs. Only HPV infections that are persistent (do not go away over many years) can lead to cervical cancer.

In 2011, more than 12,000 women in the United States are expected to be diagnosed with cervical cancer and more than

4,000 are expected to die from it. Nearly half a million women develop cervical cancer each year worldwide, and more than a quarter of a million die from it.

High-risk HPV types also cause most anal cancers. Although anal cancer is uncommon, more than 5,000 men and women in the United States are expected to be diagnosed with the disease in 2011 and 770 people are expected to die because of it.

Infection with high-risk HPV is also known to cause some cancers of the oropharynx, vulva, vagina, and penis.

Can HPV infection be prevented?

The surest way to eliminate risk for genital HPV infection is to refrain from any genital contact with another individual.

For those who are sexually active, a long-term, mutually monogamous relationship with an uninfected partner is the strategy most likely to prevent HPV infection. However, it is difficult to determine whether a partner who has been sexually active in the past is currently infected.

Research has shown that correct and consistent condom use can reduce the transmission of HPV between sexual partners. However, because areas not covered by a condom can be infected by the virus, they are unlikely to provide complete protection against transmission of infection.

The Food and Drug Administration (FDA) has approved two vaccines to prevent HPV infection: Gardasil® and Cervarix®. Both vaccines are highly effective in preventing infections with HPV types 16 and 18, two high-risk HPVs that cause about 70 percent of cervical and anal cancers. Gardasil also prevents infection with HPV types 6 and 11, which cause 90 percent of genital warts.

What are Gardasil and Cervarix?

The Gardasil vaccine is produced by Merck & Co., Inc. It is called a quadrivalent vaccine because it protects against four HPV types: 6, 11, 16, and 18. Gardasil is given through a series of three injections into muscle tissue over a 6-month period.

The FDA has approved Gardasil for use in females for the prevention of cervical cancer, and some vulvar and vaginal cancers, caused by HPV types 16 and 18, and for use in males and females for the prevention of anal cancer and precancerous anal lesions caused by HPV types 16 and 18. Gardasil is also approved for the prevention of genital warts caused by HPV types 6 and 11. The vaccine is approved for these uses in females and males ages 9 to 26.

The Cervarix vaccine is produced by GlaxoSmithKline (GSK). It is called a bivalent vaccine because it targets two

HPV types: 16 and 18. This vaccine is also given in three doses over a 6-month period. The FDA has approved Cervarix for use in females ages 9 to 25 for the prevention of cervical cancer caused by HPV types 16 and 18.

Both Gardasil and Cervarix are based on technology developed in part by NCI scientists. NCI licensed the technology to two pharmaceutical companies—Merck and GSK—to develop HPV vaccines for widespread distribution. Neither of these HPV vaccines has been proven to provide complete protection against persistent infection with other HPV types, although some initial results suggest that both vaccines might provide partial protection against a few additional HPV types that can cause cervical cancer. Overall, about 30 percent of cervical cancers will not be prevented by these vaccines. Also, in the case of Gardasil, 10 percent of genital warts will not be prevented by the vaccine. Neither vaccine prevents other sexually transmitted diseases, nor do they treat HPV infection or cervical cancer.

Because the vaccines do not protect against all HPV infections that cause cervical cancer, it is important for vaccinated women to continue to undergo cervical cancer screening. There could be some future changes in recommendations for vaccinated women.

How do HPV vaccines work?

The HPV vaccines work like other immunizations that guard against viral infections. The investigators hypothesized that the unique surface components of HPV might create an antibody response that is capable of protecting the body against infection, and that these components could be used to form the basis of a vaccine.

The HPV surface components can interact with one another to form virus-like particles (VLP) that are not infectious, because they lack DNA. However, these VLPs can attach to cells and stimulate the immune system to produce antibodies that can prevent the complete papillomavirus, in future encounters, from infecting cells.

Although HPV vaccines can help prevent future HPV infection, they do not help eliminate existing HPV infections.

How effective are the HPV vaccines?

Gardasil and Cervarix are highly effective in preventing infection with the types of HPV they target. The vaccines have been shown to provide protection against persistent cervical HPV 16/18 infections for up to 8 years, which is the maximum time of research follow-up thus far. More will be known about the total duration of protection as research continues.

HPV vaccination has also been found to prevent nearly 100 percent of the precancerous cervical cell changes that would have been caused by HPV 16/18. The data so far show duration of production for up to 6.4 years with Cervarix and for up to 5 years for Gardasil—in women who were not infected with HPV at the time of vaccination.

A recent analysis of data from a clinical trial of Cervarix found that this vaccine is just as effective at protecting women against persistent HPV 16 and 18 infection in the anus as it is at protecting them from these infections in the cervix.

Both Gardasil and Cervarix are designed to be given to people in three doses over a 6-month period. However, a recent study showed that women who received only two doses of Cervarix had just as much protection from persistent HPV 16/18 infection as women who received three doses, and the protection was observed through 4 years of follow up. Even one dose provided protection; however, these findings need to be evaluated with more research to determine whether fewer than three doses of the vaccine will provide adequate duration of protection. Nonetheless, this information may be helpful for public health officials who administer vaccination programs among groups of people unlikely to complete the three-dose regimen.

Why are these vaccines important?

Widespread vaccination has the potential to reduce cervical cancer deaths around the world by as much as two-thirds, if all women were to get the vaccine and if protection turns out to be long-term. In addition, the vaccines can reduce the need for medical care, biopsies, and invasive procedures associated with follow-up from abnormal Pap tests, thus helping to reduce health care costs and anxieties related to abnormal Pap tests and follow-up procedures.

The other cancers caused by HPV are less common than cervical cancer. However, there are no formal screening programs for these cancers, so vaccination has the potential to greatly reduce deaths from these cancers also.

How safe are the HPV vaccines?

Before any vaccine is licensed, the FDA must determine that it is both safe and effective. Both Gardasil and Cervarix have been tested in tens of thousands of people in the United States and many other countries. Thus far, no serious side effects have been shown to be caused by the vaccines. The most common problems have been brief soreness and other local symptoms at the injection site. These problems are similar to ones commonly experienced with other vaccines.

The vaccines have not been sufficiently tested during pregnancy and, therefore, should not be used by pregnant women.

A recent safety review by the FDA and the Centers for Disease Control and Prevention (CDC) considered adverse side effects related to Gardasil immunization that have been reported to the Vaccine Adverse Events Reporting System since the vaccine was licensed. The rates of adverse side effects in the safety review were consistent with what was seen in safety studies carried out before the vaccine was approved and were similar to those seen with other vaccines. However, a higher proportion of syncope (fainting) and venous thrombolic events (blood clots) were seen with Gardasil than are usually seen with other vaccines.

Falls after syncope may sometimes cause serious injuries, such as head injuries. These can largely be prevented by keeping the vaccinated person seated for up to 15 minutes after vaccination. The FDA and CDC have reminded health care providers that, to prevent falls and injuries, all vaccine recipients should remain seated or lying down and be closely observed for 15 minutes after vaccination.

Who should get these vaccines?

Both Gardasil and Cervarix are proven to be effective only if given before infection with HPV, so it is recommended that they be given before an individual is sexually active. The FDA's licensing decision includes information about the age and sex for recipients of the vaccine. The FDA has approved Gardasil for use in females and males ages 9 to 26 and Cervarix for use in females ages 9 to 25.

After a vaccine is licensed by the FDA, the Advisory Committee on Immunization Practices (ACIP) makes additional recommendations to the Secretary of the U.S. Department of Health and Human Services and the Director of the CDC on who should receive the vaccine, at what age, how often, the appropriate dose, and situations in which it should not be administered. ACIP is made up of 15 experts in fields associated with immunization.

For females, ACIP recommends that Gardasil or Cervarix vaccination be given routinely at ages 11 or 12, although the series may be started for girls as early as 9 years of age. Vaccination is also recommended for girls and women ages 13 to 26 who have not been vaccinated already or who did not complete the three-dose series. If a woman reaches the age of 26 before completing the three-dose series, ACIP recommendations say that she can still receive the remaining doses.

For males, ACIP recommends routine vaccination with Gardasil at ages 11 or 12 to prevent HPV infection. ACIP also recommends vaccinating males ages 13 to 21 who have not been vaccinated already or who did not complete the three-dose vaccination series. The vaccine may be given to males between the ages of 22 and 26.

States can decide whether or not to require vaccination of children prior to their enrollment in schools or child care. Each state makes this decision individually.

Should the vaccines be given to people who are already infected with HPV?

Although Gardasil and Cervarix have been found to be generally safe when given to people who are already infected with HPV, the vaccines do not treat infection and they provide maximum benefit if a person receives them before he or she is sexually active.

It is possible that someone infected with HPV will still get residual benefit from vaccination, even if he or she has already been infected with one or more of the types included in the vaccines. However, this possibility is still under investigation.

At present, there is no generally available test to show whether an individual has been exposed to HPV. The currently approved HPV DNA test shows only whether a person has a current HPV infection, and it identifies the HPV type. But it does not provide information on past infections.

Should women who already have cervical cell changes get the vaccines?

ACIP recommends that women who have abnormal Pap test results, which may indicate HPV infection, should still receive HPV vaccination if they are in the appropriate age group because the vaccine may protect them against high-risk HPV types that they have not yet acquired. However, these women should be told that the vaccination will not cure them of current HPV infections and that it will not treat the abnormal results of their Pap test.

Do women who have been vaccinated still need to have Pap tests?

Yes. Because these vaccines do not protect against all HPV types that can cause cancer, Pap tests continue to be essential to detect cervical cancers and precancerous changes. In addition, Pap tests are critically important for women who have not been vaccinated or who are already infected with HPV. There could be future changes in screening recommendations for vaccinated women.

What research is being done on HPV?

Researchers at NCI and elsewhere are studying how high-risk HPV types cause precancerous changes in normal cells and how these changes can be prevented or managed most efficiently. Most of this research has focused on cervical cells in women, but researchers are now investigating these questions in other tissues in which HPV may cause cancer, such as the oropharynx and anus.

NCI is conducting a community-based clinical trial of Cervarix in Costa Rica, where cervical cancer rates are high. This study is designed to obtain information about the vaccine's longer-term safety, the extent and duration of protection, the immune mechanisms of protection, and the natural history of infection with HPV types other than the types included in the vaccine.

NCI is also collaborating with other researchers on second-generation preventive vaccines and on therapeutic HPV vaccines, which would prevent the development of cancer among women previously infected with HPV. The ideal vaccine strategy would combine a preventive and therapeutic vaccine.

Another prevention strategy that is being explored is topical microbicides. Carrageenan, a compound that is extracted from a type of seaweed and used widely in foods and other products, has been found to inhibit HPV infection in laboratory studies. Clinical trials are under way to test whether a topical microbicide that contains carrageenan can prevent genital HPV infection.

Laboratory research has indicated that HPVs produce proteins known as E5, E6, and E7. These proteins interfere with the cell functions that normally prevent excessive growth. A better understanding of how these proteins interact may help researchers develop ways to interrupt the process by which HPV infection can lead to the growth of abnormal cells.

The FDA-approved tests for HPV infection in women detect viral DNA in cervical cells that are collected during a Pap test. Researchers are trying to find other ways to test for HPV infection that may be faster, more accurate, and less expensive. These new tests may be especially useful in developing countries and medically underserved populations. Researchers at NCI and elsewhere are also studying what people know and understand about HPV and cancer, the best way to communicate to the public the latest research results, and how doctors are talking with their patients about HPV. This research will help to ensure that the public receives accurate information about HPV that is easily understood and will help people get access to the appropriate tests.

Chapter 4: Pap and HPV Testing

- Cervical cancer screening, which includes the Pap test and HPV testing, is an essential part of a woman's routine health care because it can detect cancer or abnormalities that may lead to cancer of the cervix.

- Current guidelines recommend that women should have a Pap test every 3 years beginning at age 21. These guidelines further recommend that women ages 30 to 65 should have HPV and Pap cotesting every 5 years or a Pap test alone every 3 years. Women with certain risk factors may need to have more frequent screening or to continue screening beyond age 65.

- Women who have received the HPV vaccine still need regular cervical screening.

What causes cervical cancer?

Nearly all cases of cervical cancer are caused by infection with oncogenic, or high-risk, types of human papillomavirus, or HPV. There are about 12 high-risk HPV types. Infections with these sexually transmitted viruses also cause most anal cancers; many vaginal, vulvar, and penile cancers; and some oropharyngeal cancers.

Although HPV infection is very common, most infections will be suppressed by the immune system within 1 to 2 years without causing cancer. These transient infections may cause temporary changes in cervical cells. If a cervical infection with a high-risk HPV type persists, the cellular changes can eventually develop into more severe precancerous lesions. If precancerous lesions are not treated, they can progress to cancer. It can take 10 to 20 years or more for a persistent infection with a high-risk HPV type to develop into cancer.

What is cervical cancer screening?

Cervical cancer screening is an essential part of a woman's routine health care. It is a way to detect abnormal cervical cells, including precancerous cervical lesions, as well as early cervical cancers. Both precancerous lesions and early cervical cancers can be treated very successfully. Routine cervical screening has been shown to greatly reduce both the number of new cervical cancers diagnosed each year and deaths from the disease.

Cervical cancer screening includes two types of screening tests: cytology-based screening, known as the Pap test or Pap smear, and HPV testing. The main purpose of screening with the Pap test is to detect abnormal cells that may develop into cancer if left untreated. The Pap test can also find noncancerous conditions, such as infections and inflammation. It can also find cancer cells. In regularly screened populations, the Pap test identifies most abnormal cells before they become cancer.

HPV testing is used to look for the presence of DNA or RNA from high-risk HPV types in cervical cells. These tests can sometimes detect HPV infections before cell abnormalities are evident. The most common test detects DNA from the high-risk HPV types, but it cannot identify the specific type or types that are present. Another test is specific for DNA from HPV types 16 and 18, the two types that cause most HPV-associated cancers. A third test can detect DNA from several high-risk HPV types and can indicate whether HPV-16 or HPV-18 is present. A fourth test detects RNA from the most common high-risk HPV types.

How is cervical cancer screening done?

Cervical cancer screening can be done in a medical office, a clinic, or a hospital. It is often done during a pelvic examination.

While a woman lies on an exam table, a health care professional inserts an instrument called a speculum into her vagina to widen it so that the upper portion of the vagina and the cervix can be seen. This procedure also allows the health care professional to take a sample of cervical cells. The cells are taken with a wooden or plastic scraper and/or a cervical brush and are then prepared for analysis in one of two ways. In a conventional Pap test, the specimen (or smear) is placed on a glass microscope slide and a fixative is added. In an automated liquid-based Pap cytology test, cervical cells collected with a brush or other instrument are placed in a vial of liquid preservative. The slide or vial is then sent to a laboratory for analysis.

In the United States, automated liquid-based Pap cytology testing has largely replaced conventional Pap tests. One advantage of liquid-based testing is that the same cell sample can also be tested for the presence of high-risk types of HPV, a process known as "Pap and HPV cotesting." In addition, liquid-based cytology appears to reduce the likelihood of an unsatisfactory specimen. However, conventional and liquid-based Pap tests appear to have a similar ability to detect cellular abnormalities.

<u>When should a woman begin cervical cancer screening, and how often should she be screened?</u>

Women should talk with their doctor about when to start screening and how often to be screened. In March 2012, updated screening guidelines were released by the United States Preventive Services Task Force and jointly by the American Cancer Society, the American Society for Colposcopy and Cervical Pathology, and the American Society for Clinical Pathology. These guidelines recommend that women have their first Pap test at age 21. Although previous guidelines recommended that women have their first Pap test 3 years after they start having sexual intercourse, waiting until age 21 is now recommended because adolescents have a very low risk of cervical cancer and a high likelihood that cervical cell abnormalities will go away on their own. According to the updated guidelines, women ages 21 through 29 should be screened with a Pap test every 3 years. Women ages 30 through 65 can then be screened every 5 years with Pap and HPV cotesting or every 3 years with a Pap test alone.

The guidelines advise that routine Pap and HPV cotesting be limited to women age 30 and older because transient HPV infections are very common among women in their twenties. Including routine HPV testing in cervical screening of younger women would detect many infections that will be suppressed by the immune system and not lead to cancer. In older women, HPV infections are more likely to represent persistent infections—that is, infections that have the potential to progress to cervical cancer if not detected or treated. However, HPV testing can be used in women of any age to help clarify unclear Pap test findings and help doctors decide if further evaluation is needed.

The guidelines also note that women with certain risk factors may need to have more frequent screening or to continue screening beyond age 65. These risk factors include being infected with the human immunodeficiency virus (HIV), being immunosuppressed, having been exposed to diethylstilbestrol before birth, and having been treated for a precancerous cervical lesion or cervical cancer.

Women who have had a hysterectomy (surgery to remove the uterus and cervix) do not need to have cervical screening, unless the hysterectomy was done to treat a precancerous cervical lesion or cervical cancer.

What are the benefits of Pap and HPV cotesting?

For women age 30 and older, Pap and HPV cotesting is less likely to miss an abnormality (i.e., has a lower false-negative rate) than Pap testing alone. Therefore, a woman with a negative HPV test and normal Pap test has very little risk of a serious abnormality developing over the next several years.

In fact, researchers have found that, when Pap and HPV cotesting is used, lengthening the screening interval to 5 years still allows abnormalities to be detected in time to treat them, but it reduces the detection of transient HPV infections.

Adding HPV testing to Pap testing may also improve the detection of glandular cell abnormalities, including adenocarcinoma of the cervix (cancer of the glandular cells of the cervix). Glandular cells are mucus-producing cells found in the endocervical canal (the opening in the center of the cervix) or in the lining of the uterus. Glandular cell abnormalities and adenocarcinoma of the cervix are much less common than squamous cell abnormalities and squamous cell carcinoma. There is some evidence that Pap testing is not as good at detecting adenocarcinoma and glandular cell abnormalities as it is at detecting squamous cell abnormalities and cancers.

Can HPV testing be used alone for cervical cancer screening?

Not enough data are available to determine whether HPV testing can be used alone to screen for cervical cancer. Ongoing studies are investigating the possibility of using routine HPV testing as a primary screening method, with follow-up testing by a Pap test or other tests for women who test positive for a high-risk HPV type.

What is the best time to be screened for cervical cancer?

The best time for a woman to have cervical screening is between 10 and 20 days after the first day of her last menstrual period. A woman should not have cervical screening when she is menstruating. For about 2 days before the test, she should avoid sexual intercourse, douching, or using vaginal medicines or spermicidal foams, creams, or jellies (except as directed by a doctor) because they may wash away or hide abnormal cells. After the test, she can go back to her normal activities and return to work right away.

How are the results of Pap tests reported?

A doctor may simply describe Pap test results to a patient as "normal" or "abnormal." It is important to remember that abnormalities rarely become cancerous, and even severe lesions do not always lead to cancer. Likewise, HPV test results can either be "positive," meaning that a patient is infected with at least one high-risk HPV type, or "negative," indicating that high-risk HPV types were not found. A woman may want to ask her doctor for specific information about her Pap and HPV test results and what these results mean.

Most laboratories in the United States use a standard set of terms, called the Bethesda System, to report Pap test results. Under the Bethesda System, samples that have no cell abnormalities are reported as "negative for intraepithelial lesion or malignancy." A negative Pap test report may also note certain benign (non-neoplastic) findings, such as common infections or inflammation. Pap test results also indicate whether the specimen was satisfactory or unsatisfactory for examination.

The Bethesda System considers abnormalities of squamous cells and glandular cells separately. Squamous cell abnormalities are divided into the following categories, ranging from the mildest to the most severe.

- *Atypical squamous cells (ASC)* are the most common abnormal finding in Pap tests. The Bethesda System divides this category into two groups, which are described below.
  - *ASC-US*: atypical squamous cells of undetermined significance. The squamous cells do not appear completely normal, but doctors are uncertain about what the cell changes mean. Sometimes the changes are

related to an HPV infection, but they can also be caused by other factors. For women who have ASC-US, a sample of cells may be tested for the presence of high-risk HPV types. If high-risk HPV type is present, follow-up testing will usually be performed. On the other hand, a negative HPV test can provide reassurance that cancer or a precancerous condition is not present.

- ○ *ASC-H*: atypical squamous cells, cannot exclude a high-grade squamous intraepithelial lesion. The cells do not appear normal, but doctors are uncertain about what the cell changes mean. ASC-H lesions may be at higher risk of being precancerous compared with ASC-US lesions.

- *Low-grade squamous intraepithelial lesions (LSILs)* are considered mild abnormalities caused by HPV infection. Low-grade means that there are early changes in the size and shape of cells. Intraepithelial refers to the layer of cells that forms the surface of the cervix. LSILs are sometimes classified as mild dysplasia. LSILs may also be classified as cervical intraepithelial neoplasia (CIN-1).

- *High-grade squamous intraepithelial lesions (HSILs)* are more severe abnormalities that have a higher likelihood of progressing to cancer if left untreated. High-grade means that there are more evident changes in the size and shape of the abnormal (precancerous) cells and that the cells look very different from normal cells. HSILs include lesions with moderate or severe dysplasia and carcinoma in situ (CIS). HSIL lesions are sometimes classified as CIN-2, CIN-3, or CIN-2/3. CIS is commonly included in the CIN-3 category.

- *Squamous cell carcinoma* is cervical cancer. The abnormal squamous cells have invaded deeper into the cervix or into other tissues or organs. In a well-screened population, such as that in the United States, a finding of cancer during cervical screening is extremely rare.

Glandular cell abnormalities are divided into the following categories:

- *Atypical glandular cells (AGC),* meaning the glandular cells do not appear normal, but doctors are uncertain about what the cell changes mean.
- *Endocervical adenocarcinoma in situ (AIS),* meaning that precancerous cells are found only in glandular tissue of the cervix.
- *Adenocarcinoma* includes not only cancer of the endocervical canal itself but also, in some cases, endometrial, extrauterine, and other cancers.

What follow-up tests are done if cervical cancer screening results are abnormal?

If a woman receiving Pap and HPV cotesting is found to have a normal Pap test result with a positive HPV test that detects the group of high-risk HPV types, the doctor will probably have the woman return in a year for repeat screening to see if the HPV infection persists and whether any cell changes have developed that need further follow-up. Alternatively, the woman may have another HPV test that looks specifically for HPV-16 and HPV-18, the two HPV types that cause most cervical cancers. If either of these types is present, a woman will likely have follow-up testing.

If a woman is found to have an ASC-US Pap test result, her doctor may have the sample tested for high-risk HPV types or may repeat the Pap test to determine whether further follow-up is needed. Many times, cell changes in the cervix go away without treatment, especially if there is no evidence of infection with high-risk HPV. Doctors may prescribe estrogen cream for women with ASC-US who are near or past menopause. Because ASC-US cell changes can be caused by low hormone levels, applying an estrogen cream to the cervix for a few weeks can usually help to clarify their cause.

Follow-up testing for ASC-US with a positive HPV test, for LSIL, or for HSIL, may involve a colposcopy, in which an instrument much like a microscope (called a colposcope) is used to examine the vagina and the cervix. During a colposcopy, the doctor inserts a speculum to widen the vagina and may apply a dilute vinegar solution to the cervix, which causes abnormal areas to turn white. The doctor then uses the colposcope (which remains outside the body) to observe the cervix.

If abnormal tissue is found during a colposcopy, the doctor may perform endocervical curettage or a biopsy. A biopsy is the removal of cells or tissues from the abnormal area for examination under a microscope. Endocervical curettage is a type of biopsy that involves scraping cells from inside the endocervical canal with a small spoon-shaped tool called a curette.

If follow-up testing shows cells with more severe abnormalities, further treatment is needed. Without treatment, these cells may turn into cancer. Treatment options include the following:

- LEEP (loop electrosurgical excision procedure) uses an electrical current that is passed through a thin wire loop to act as a knife to remove tissue.
- Cryotherapy destroys abnormal tissue by freezing it.
- Laser therapy uses a narrow beam of intense light to destroy or remove abnormal cells.
- Conization removes a cone-shaped piece of tissue using a knife, a laser, or the LEEP technique.

Do women who have been vaccinated against HPVs still need to be screened for cervical cancer?

Yes. Because current HPV vaccines do not protect against all HPV types that cause cervical cancer, it is important for vaccinated women to continue to undergo routine cervical cancer screening.

What are the limitations of cervical cancer screening?

Like any screening test, cervical cancer screening is not completely accurate. Sometimes a patient can be told that she has abnormal cells when the cells are actually normal (a false-positive result), or she can be told that her cells are normal when in fact there is an abnormality that was not detected (a false-negative result).

Cervical cancer screening has another limitation, caused by the nature of HPV infections. Because most HPV infections are transient and produce only temporary changes in cervical cells, overly frequent cervical screening could detect cervical cell changes that would never cause cancer. Treating abnormalities that would have gone away on their own can cause needless psychological stress. In addition, follow-up tests and treatments can be uncomfortable, and some treatments that remove cervical tissue, such as LEEP and conization, have the potential to weaken the cervix and may affect fertility or slightly increase the rate of premature delivery, depending on how much tissue is removed.

The screening intervals in the 2012 guidelines are intended to minimize the harms caused by treating abnormalities that would never progress to cancer while also limiting false-negative results that would delay the diagnosis and treatment of a precancerous condition or cancer. With these intervals, if an HPV infection or abnormal cells are missed at one screen, chances are good that abnormal cells will be detected at the next screening exam, when they can still be treated successfully.

Chapter 5: Preventive Mastectomy

- Preventive mastectomy (also called prophylactic or risk-reducing mastectomy) is the surgical removal of one or both breasts. It is done to prevent or reduce the risk of breast cancer in women who are at high risk of developing the disease.

- Existing data suggest that preventive mastectomy may significantly reduce (by about 90 percent) the chance of developing breast cancer in moderate- and high-risk women.

- It is important for a woman who is considering preventive mastectomy to talk with a doctor about her risk of developing breast cancer, the surgical procedure and its potential complications, and alternatives to surgery.

- Many women who choose to have preventive mastectomy also decide to have breast reconstruction to restore the shape of the breast.

What is preventive mastectomy, and what types of procedures are used in preventive mastectomy?

Preventive mastectomy (also called prophylactic or risk-reducing mastectomy) is the surgical removal of one or both breasts in an effort to prevent or reduce the risk of breast cancer. Preventive mastectomy involves one of two basic procedures: total mastectomy and subcutaneous mastectomy. In a total mastectomy, the doctor removes the entire breast and nipple. In a subcutaneous mastectomy, the doctor removes the breast tissue but leaves the nipple intact. Doctors most often recommend a total mastectomy because it removes more tissue than a subcutaneous mastectomy. A total mastectomy provides the greatest protection against cancer developing in any remaining breast tissue.

Why would a woman consider undergoing preventive mastectomy?

Women who are at high risk of developing breast cancer may consider preventive mastectomy as a way of decreasing their risk of this disease. Some of the factors that increase a woman's chance of developing breast cancer are listed below.

- *Previous breast cancer*—A woman who has had cancer in one breast is more likely to develop a new cancer in the opposite breast. Occasionally, such women may consider preventive mastectomy to decrease the chance of developing a new breast cancer.

- *Family history of breast cancer*—Preventive mastectomy may be an option for a woman whose mother, sister, or daughter had breast cancer, especially if they were diagnosed before age 50. If multiple family members have breast or ovarian cancer, then a woman's risk of breast cancer may be even higher.

- *Breast cancer-causing gene alteration*—A woman who tests positive for changes, or mutations, in certain genes that increase the risk of breast cancer (such as the BRCA1 or BRCA2 gene) may consider preventive mastectomy.

- *Lobular carcinoma in situ*—Preventive mastectomy is sometimes considered for a woman with lobular carcinoma in situ, a condition that increases the risk of developing breast cancer in either breast.

- *Diffuse and indeterminate breast microcalcifications or dense breasts*—Rarely, preventive mastectomy may be considered for a woman who has diffuse and indeterminate breast microcalcifications (tiny deposits of calcium in the breast) or for a woman whose breast tissue is very dense. Dense breast tissue is linked to an increased risk of breast cancer and also makes diagnosing breast abnormalities difficult. Multiple biopsies, which may be necessary for diagnosing abnormalities in dense breasts, cause scarring and further complicate examination of the breast tissue, by both physical examination and mammography.

- *Radiation therapy*—A woman who had radiation therapy to the chest (including the breasts) before age 30 is at an increased risk of developing breast cancer throughout her life. This includes women treated for Hodgkin lymphoma.

It is important for a woman who is considering preventive mastectomy to talk with a doctor about her risk of developing breast cancer (with or without a mastectomy), the surgical procedure, and potential complications. All women are different, so preventive mastectomy should be considered in the context of each woman's unique risk factors and her level of concern.

How effective is preventive mastectomy in preventing or reducing the risk of breast cancer?

Existing data suggest that preventive mastectomy may significantly reduce (by about 90 percent) the chance of developing breast cancer in moderate- and high-risk women. However, no one can be certain that this procedure will protect an individual woman from breast cancer. Breast tissue is widely distributed on the chest wall, and can sometimes be found in the armpit, above the collarbone, and as far down as the abdomen. Because it is impossible for a surgeon to remove all breast tissue, breast cancer can still develop in the small amount of remaining tissue.

What are the possible drawbacks of preventive mastectomy?

Like any other surgery, complications such as bleeding or infection can occur. Preventive mastectomy is irreversible and can have psychological effects on a woman due to a change in body image and loss of normal breast functions. A woman should discuss her feelings about mastectomy, as well as alternatives to surgery, with her health care providers. Some women obtain a second medical opinion to help with the decision.

What alternatives to surgery exist for preventing or reducing the risk of breast cancer?

Doctors do not always agree on the most effective way to manage the care of women who have a strong family history of breast cancer and/or have other risk factors for the disease. Some doctors may advise very close monitoring (periodic mammograms, regular checkups that include a clinical breast examination performed by a health care professional, and monthly breast self-examinations) to increase the chance of detecting breast cancer at an early stage. Some doctors may recommend preventive mastectomy, while others may prescribe tamoxifen or raloxifene, medications that have been shown to decrease the chances of getting breast cancer in women at high risk of the disease.

Doctors may also encourage women at high risk to limit their consumption of alcohol, eat a low-fat diet, engage in regular exercise, and avoid menopausal hormone use. Although these lifestyle recommendations make sense and are part of an overall healthy way of living, we do not yet have clear and convincing proof that they specifically reduce the risk of developing breast cancer.

What is breast reconstruction?

Breast reconstruction is a plastic surgery procedure in which the shape of the breast is rebuilt. Many women who choose to have preventive mastectomy also decide to have breast reconstruction, either at the time of the mastectomy or at some later time.

Before performing breast reconstruction, the plastic surgeon carefully examines the breasts and discusses the reconstruction options. In one type of reconstructive procedure, the surgeon inserts an implant (a balloon-like device filled with saline or silicone) under the skin and the chest muscles. Another procedure, called tissue flap reconstruction, uses skin, fat, and muscle from the woman's abdomen, back, or buttocks to create the breast shape. The surgeon will discuss with the patient any limitations on exercise or arm motion that might result from these operations.

What type of follow-up care is needed after reconstructive surgery?

Women who have reconstructive surgery are monitored carefully to detect and treat complications, such as infection, movement of the implant, or contracture (the formation of a firm, fibrous shell or scar tissue around the implant caused by the body's reaction to the implant). Women who have tissue flap reconstruction may want to ask their surgeon about physical therapy, which can help them adjust to limitations in activity and exercise after surgery. Routine screening for breast cancer is also part of the postoperative follow-up, because the risk of cancer cannot be completely eliminated. When women with breast implants have mammograms, they should tell the radiology technician about the implant. Special procedures may be necessary to improve the accuracy of the mammogram and to avoid damaging the implant. However, women who have had reconstructive surgery on both breasts should ask their doctors whether mammograms are still necessary.

Chapter 6: Antioxidants and Cancer Prevention

- Antioxidants protect cells from damage caused by unstable molecules known as free radicals.

- Laboratory and animal research have shown that antioxidants help prevent the free radical damage that is associated with cancer. However, results from recent studies in people (clinical trials) are not consistent.

- Antioxidants are provided by a healthy diet that includes a variety of fruits and vegetables.

What are antioxidants?

Antioxidants are substances that may protect cells from the damage caused by unstable molecules known as free radicals. Free radical damage may lead to cancer. Antioxidants interact with and stabilize free radicals and may prevent some of the damage free radicals might otherwise cause. Examples of antioxidants include beta-carotene, lycopene, vitamins C, E, and A, and other substances.

Can antioxidants prevent cancer?

Considerable laboratory evidence from chemical, cell culture, and animal studies indicates that antioxidants may slow or possibly prevent the development of cancer. However, information from recent clinical trials is less clear. In recent years, large-scale, randomized clinical trials reached inconsistent conclusions.

What was shown in previously published large-scale clinical trials?

Five large-scale clinical trials published in the 1990s reached differing conclusions about the effect of antioxidants on cancer. The studies examined the effect of beta-carotene and other antioxidants on cancer in different patient groups. However, beta-carotene appeared to have different effects depending upon the patient population. The conclusions of each study are summarized below.

- The first large randomized trial on antioxidants and cancer risk was the Chinese Cancer Prevention Study, published in 1993. This trial investigated the effect of a combination of beta-carotene, vitamin E, and selenium on cancer in healthy Chinese men and women at high risk for gastric cancer. The study showed a combination of beta-carotene, vitamin E, and selenium significantly reduced incidence of both gastric cancer and cancer overall.

- A 1994 cancer prevention study entitled the Alpha-Tocopherol (vitamin E)/ Beta-Carotene Cancer Prevention Study (ATBC) demonstrated that lung cancer rates of Finnish male smokers increased significantly with beta-carotene and were not affected by vitamin E.
- Another 1994 study, the Beta-Carotene and Retinol (vitamin A) Efficacy Trial (CARET), also demonstrated a possible increase in lung cancer associated with antioxidants.
- The 1996 Physicians' Health Study I (PHS) found no change in cancer rates associated with beta-carotene and aspirin taken by U.S. male physicians.
- The 1999 Women's Health Study (WHS) tested effects of vitamin E and beta-carotene in the prevention of cancer and cardiovascular disease among women age 45 years or older. Among apparently healthy women, there was no benefit or harm from beta-carotene supplementation. Investigation of the effect of vitamin E is ongoing.

Are antioxidants under investigation in current large-scale clinical trials?

Three large-scale clinical trials continue to investigate the effect of antioxidants on cancer. The objective of each of these studies is described below.

- The Women's Health Study (WHS) is currently evaluating the effect of vitamin E in the primary prevention of cancer among U.S. female health professionals age 45 and older. The WHS is expected to conclude in August 2004.

- The Selenium and Vitamin E Cancer Prevention Trial (SELECT) is taking place in the United States, Puerto Rico, and Canada. SELECT is trying to find out if taking selenium and/or vitamin E supplements can prevent prostate cancer in men age 50 or older. The SELECT trial is expected to stop recruiting patients in May 2006.

- The Physicians' Health Study II (PHS II) is a follow up to the earlier clinical trial by the same name. The study is investigating the effects of vitamin E, C, and multivitamins on prostate

cancer and total cancer incidence. The PHS II is
expected to conclude in August 2007.

How might antioxidants prevent cancer?

Antioxidants neutralize free radicals as the natural by-
product of normal cell processes. Free radicals are molecules
with incomplete electron shells which make them more
chemically reactive than those with complete electron shells.
Exposure to various environmental factors, including tobacco
smoke and radiation, can also lead to free radical formation.
In humans, the most common form of free radicals is oxygen.
When an oxygen molecule ($O2$) becomes electrically charged
or "radicalized" it tries to steal electrons from other
molecules, causing damage to the DNA and other molecules.
Over time, such damage may become irreversible and lead to
disease including cancer. Antioxidants are often described as
"mopping up" free radicals, meaning they neutralize the
electrical charge and prevent the free radical from taking
electrons from other molecules.

Which foods are rich in antioxidants?

Antioxidants are abundant in fruits and vegetables, as well as
in other foods including nuts, grains, and some meats,

poultry, and fish. The list below describes food sources of common antioxidants.

- *Beta-carotene* is found in many foods that are orange in color, including sweet potatoes, carrots, cantaloupe, squash, apricots, pumpkin, and mangos. Some green, leafy vegetables, including collard greens, spinach, and kale, are also rich in beta-carotene.
- *Lutein*, best known for its association with healthy eyes, is abundant in green, leafy vegetables such as collard greens, spinach, and kale.
- *Lycopene* is a potent antioxidant found in tomatoes, watermelon, guava, papaya, apricots, pink grapefruit, blood oranges, and other foods. Estimates suggest 85 percent of American dietary intake of lycopene comes from tomatoes and tomato products.
- *Selenium* is a mineral, not an antioxidant nutrient. However, it is a component of antioxidant enzymes. Plant foods like rice and wheat are the major dietary sources of selenium in most countries. The amount of selenium in soil, which varies by region,

determines the amount of selenium in the foods grown in that soil. Animals that eat grains or plants grown in selenium-rich soil have higher levels of selenium in their muscle. In the United States, meats and bread are common sources of dietary selenium. Brazil nuts also contain large quantities of selenium.

- *Vitamin A* is found in three main forms: retinol (Vitamin A1), 3,4-didehydroretinol (Vitamin A2), and 3-hydroxy-retinol (Vitamin A3). Foods rich in vitamin A include liver, sweet potatoes, carrots, milk, egg yolks, and mozzarella cheese.

- *Vitamin C* is also called ascorbic acid, and can be found in high abundance in many fruits and vegetables and is also found in cereals, beef, poultry, and fish.

- *Vitamin E*, also known as alpha-tocopherol, is found in almonds, in many oils including wheat germ, safflower, corn, and soybean oils, and is also found in mangos, nuts, broccoli, and other foods.

Chapter 7: Cruciferous Vegetables and Cancer Prevention

- Cruciferous vegetables contain vitamins, minerals, other nutrients, and chemicals known as glucosinolates.
- Glucosinolates break down into several biologically active compounds that are being studied for possible anticancer effects.
- Some of these compounds have shown anticancer effects in cells and animals, but the results of studies with humans have been less clear.

What are cruciferous vegetables?

Cruciferous vegetables are part of the Brassica genus of plants. They include the following vegetables, among others:

- Arugula
- Bok choy
- Broccoli
- Brussels sprouts
- Cabbage
- Cauliflower
- Collard greens

- Horseradish
- Kale
- Radishes
- Rutabaga
- Turnips
- Watercress
- Wasabi

Why are cancer researchers studying cruciferous vegetables?

Cruciferous vegetables are rich in nutrients, including several carotenoids (beta-carotene, lutein, zeaxanthin); vitamins C, E, and K; folate; and minerals. They also are a good fiber source.

In addition, cruciferous vegetables contain a group of substances known as glucosinolates, which are sulfur-containing chemicals. These chemicals are responsible for the pungent aroma and bitter flavor of cruciferous vegetables. During food preparation, chewing, and digestion, the glucosinolates in cruciferous vegetables are broken down to form biologically active compounds such as indoles, nitriles, thiocyanates, and isothiocyanates. Indole-3-carbinol (an indole) and sulforaphane (an isothiocyanate) have been most frequently examined for their anticancer effects.

Indoles and isothiocyanates have been found to inhibit the development of cancer in several organs in rats and mice, including the bladder, breast, colon, liver, lung, and stomach. Studies in animals and experiments with cells grown in the laboratory have identified several potential ways in which these compounds may help prevent cancer:

- They help protect cells from DNA damage.
- They help inactivate carcinogens.
- They have antiviral and antibacterial effects.
- They have anti-inflammatory effects.
- They induce cell death (apoptosis).
- They inhibit tumor blood vessel formation (angiogenesis) and tumor cell migration (needed for metastasis).

Studies in humans, however, have shown mixed results.

Is there evidence that cruciferous vegetables can help reduce cancer risk in people?

Researchers have investigated possible associations between intake of cruciferous vegetables and the risk of cancer. The evidence has been reviewed by various experts. Key studies regarding four common forms of cancer are described briefly below.

- Prostate cancer: Cohort studies in the Netherlands, United States, and Europe have examined a wide range of daily cruciferous vegetable intakes and found little or no association with prostate cancer risk. However, some case-control studies have found that people who ate greater amounts of cruciferous vegetables had a lower risk of prostate cancer.
- Colorectal cancer: Cohort studies in the United States and the Netherlands have generally found no association between cruciferous vegetable intake and colorectal cancer risk. The exception is one study in the Netherlands—the Netherlands Cohort Study on Diet and Cancer—in which women (but not men) who had a high intake of cruciferous vegetables had a reduced risk of colon (but not rectal) cancer.
- Lung cancer: Cohort studies in Europe, the Netherlands, and the United States have had varying results. Most studies have reported little association, but one U.S. analysis—using data from the Nurses' Health Study and the Health Professionals' Follow-up Study—showed that women who ate more than 5 servings of

cruciferous vegetables per week had a lower risk
of lung cancer.

- Breast cancer: One case-control study found that
women who ate greater amounts of cruciferous
vegetables had a lower risk of breast cancer. A
meta-analysis of studies conducted in the United
States, Canada, Sweden, and the Netherlands
found no association between cruciferous
vegetable intake and breast cancer risk. An
additional cohort study of women in the United
States similarly showed only a weak association
with breast cancer risk.

A few studies have shown that the bioactive components of
cruciferous vegetables can have beneficial effects on
biomarkers of cancer-related processes in people. For
example, one study found that indole-3-carbinol was more
effective than placebo in reducing the growth of abnormal
cells on the surface of the cervix.

In addition, several case-control studies have shown that
specific forms of the gene that encodes glutathione S-
transferase, which is the enzyme that metabolizes and helps
eliminate isothiocyanates from the body, may influence the
association between cruciferous vegetable intake and human
lung and colorectal cancer risk.

Are cruciferous vegetables part of a healthy diet?

The federal government's <u>Dietary Guidelines for Americans 2010</u> recommend consuming a variety of vegetables each day. Different vegetables are rich in different nutrients. Vegetables are categorized into five subgroups: dark-green, red and orange, beans and peas (legumes), starchy, and other vegetables. Cruciferous vegetables fall into the "dark-green vegetables" category and the "other vegetables" category. Higher consumption of vegetables in general may protect against some diseases, including some types of cancer. However, when researchers try to distinguish cruciferous vegetables from other foods in the diet, it can be challenging to get clear results because study participants may have trouble remembering precisely what they ate. Also, people who eat cruciferous vegetables may be more likely than people who don't to have other healthy behaviors that reduce disease risk. It is also possible that some people, because of their genetic background, metabolize dietary isothiocyanates differently. However, research has not yet revealed a specific group of people who, because of their genetics, benefit more than other people from eating cruciferous vegetables.

Chapter 8: Garlic and Cancer Prevention

What is garlic?

Garlic is a vegetable (Allium sativum) that belongs to the Allium class of bulb-shaped plants, which also includes onions, chives, leeks, and scallions. Garlic is used for flavoring in cooking and is unique because of its high sulfur content. In addition to sulfur, garlic also contains arginine, oligosaccharides, flavonoids, and selenium, all of which may be beneficial to health.

The characteristic odor and flavor of garlic comes from sulfur compounds formed from allicin, the major precursor of garlic's bioactive compounds, which are formed when garlic bulbs are chopped, crushed, or damaged. Bioactive compounds are defined as substances in foods or dietary supplements, other than those needed to meet basic nutritional needs, that are responsible for changes in health status.

What are the types of garlic preparations?

Garlic supplements can be classified into four groups: Garlic essential oil, garlic oil macerate, garlic powder, and garlic extract.

- Garlic essential oil is obtained by passing steam through garlic. Commercially available garlic oil capsules generally contain vegetable oil, but only have a small amount of garlic essential oil because of its strong odor.
- Garlic oil macerate products are made from encapsulated mixtures of whole garlic cloves ground into vegetable oil.
- Garlic powder is produced by slicing or crushing garlic cloves, then drying and grinding them into powder. Garlic powder is used as a flavoring agent for condiments and food and is thought to retain the same ingredients as raw garlic.
- Garlic extract is made from whole or sliced garlic cloves that are soaked in an alcohol solution (an extracting solution) for varying amounts of time. Powdered forms of the extract also are available

Do findings from population studies offer evidence that garlic may prevent cancer?

Several population studies show an association between increased intake of garlic and reduced risk of certain cancers, including cancers of the stomach, colon, esophagus, pancreas, and breast. Population studies are multidisciplinary studies of population groups that investigate the cause, incidence, or spread of a disease or examine the effect of health-related interventions, dietary and nutritional intakes, or environmental exposures. An analysis of data from seven population studies showed that the higher the amount of raw and cooked garlic consumed, the lower the risk of stomach and colorectal cancer.

The European Prospective Investigation into Cancer and Nutrition (EPIC) is an ongoing multinational study involving men and women from 10 different countries. This study is investigating the effects of nutrition on cancer. In the study, higher intakes of onion and garlic were associated with a reduced risk of intestinal cancer.

The Iowa Women's Study is a large prospective study investigating whether diet, distribution of body fat, and other risk factors are related to cancer incidence in older women. Findings from the study showed a strong association between garlic consumption and colon cancer risk. Women who consumed the highest amounts of garlic had a 50 percent lower risk of cancer of the distal colon compared with women who had the lowest level of garlic consumption.

Several population studies conducted in China centered on garlic consumption and cancer risk. In one study, investigators found that frequent consumption of garlic and various types of onions and chives was associated with reduced risk of esophageal and stomach cancers, with greater risk reductions seen for higher levels of consumption. Similarly, in another study, the consumption of allium vegetables, especially garlic and onions, was linked to a reduced risk of stomach cancer. In a third study, greater intake of allium vegetables (more than 10 g per day vs. less than 2.2 g per day), particularly garlic and scallions, was associated with an approximately 50 percent reduction in prostate cancer risk.

Evidence also suggests that increased garlic consumption may reduce pancreatic cancer risk. A study conducted in the San Francisco Bay area found that pancreatic cancer risk was 54 percent lower in people who ate larger amounts of garlic compared with those who ate lower amounts.

In addition, a study in France found that increased garlic consumption was associated with a statistically significant reduction in breast cancer risk. After considering total calorie intake and other established risk factors, breast cancer risk was reduced in those consuming greater amounts of fiber, garlic, and onions.

Do findings from clinical trials offer evidence that garlic may prevent cancer?

Few clinical trials (research studies with people) have been done to examine the potential anticancer effects of garlic. Three randomized clinical trials have evaluated the effect of garlic intake on gastric cancer risk. In one study, which involved over 5,000 Chinese men and women at high risk for stomach cancer, researchers compared the effects of taking a combination of 200 mg synthetic allitridum (an extract of garlic used as a medicine in China for over 3,000 years) daily and 100 micrograms selenium every other day with taking a placebo (an inactive substance or treatment that looks the same as, and is given the same way as, an active drug or treatment being tested) for 5 years. In the group that received allitridum and selenium, the risk for all tumors combined was reduced by 33 percent and the risk for stomach cancer was reduced by 52 percent in comparison with the group that received only the placebo.

In contrast, findings from another randomized trial involving individuals with precancerous stomach lesions found that garlic supplementation (800 mg garlic extract plus 4 mg steam-distilled garlic oil daily) did not improve the prevalence (number of existing cases) of precancerous gastric lesions or reduce the incidence (number of new cases) of gastric cancer.

A third randomized study in Japan compared the effects of daily high-dose (2.4 mL) and low-dose (0.16 mL) intake of aged-garlic extract after 6 and 12 months of use on individuals with colorectal adenomas (noncancerous tumors). At the end of 12 months, 67 percent of the low-intake group developed new adenomas compared with 47 percent in the high-intake group.

The results of a small, nonrandomized study indicate that the application of garlic extracts to some skin tumors may be beneficial. In the study, which involved 21 persons with basal cell carcinoma, the application of ajoene (a sulfurous chemical found in garlic) to the skin for 1 month markedly decreased the size of 17 tumors, increased tumor size in 3 patients, and resulted in no change in 1 other patient. Changes in tumor size ranged from an 88 percent reduction to a 69 percent increase, with an overall median reduction of 47 percent.

What are the current issues and controversies surrounding the use of garlic in cancer prevention?

Study limitations, including the accuracy of reporting the amounts and frequency of garlic consumed, and the inability to compare data from studies that used different garlic products and amounts make an overall conclusion about garlic and cancer prevention extremely difficult. Since many of the studies looking at garlic use and cancer prevention have used multi-ingredient products, it is unclear whether garlic alone or in combination with other nutritional components may have the greatest effect.

Well-designed dietary studies in humans using predetermined amounts of garlic (intervention studies) are needed to determine potentially effective intakes. Studies directly comparing various garlic preparations are also needed.

How might garlic act to prevent cancer?

Protective effects from garlic may arise from its antibacterial properties or from its ability to block the formation of cancer-causing substances, halt the activation of cancer-causing substances, enhance DNA repair, reduce cell proliferation, or induce cell death.

How much garlic may be useful for cancer prevention?

The National Cancer Institute, part of the National Institutes of Health, does not recommend any dietary supplement for the prevention of cancer, but recognizes garlic as one of several vegetables with potential anticancer properties. Because all garlic preparations are not the same, it is difficult to determine the exact amount of garlic that may be needed to reduce cancer risk. Furthermore, the active compounds present in garlic may lose their effectiveness with time, handling, and processing. The World Health Organization's (WHO) guidelines for general health promotion for adults is a daily dose of 2 to 5 g of fresh garlic (approximately one clove), 0.4 to 1.2 g of dried garlic powder, 2 to 5 mg of garlic oil, 300 to 1,000 mg of garlic extract, or other formulations that are equal to 2 to 5 mg of allicin.

What are the safety considerations?

Although garlic has been used safely in cooking, excessive consumption can cause some side effects, in addition to strong breath and body odors. Garlic occasionally causes allergies that can range from mild irritation to potentially life-threatening problems. Ingestion of fresh garlic bulbs, extracts, or oil on an empty stomach may occasionally cause heartburn, nausea, vomiting, and diarrhea. Some animal and human studies suggest that garlic can lower blood sugar levels and increase insulin.

Garlic has been shown to interfere with several prescription drugs, especially the HIV medication saquinavir (brand names Invirase® and Fortovase®). Garlic can lower the serum levels of saquinavir by as much as 50 percent. Garlic also acts as a natural blood thinner and, thus, should be avoided by pregnant women, people about to undergo surgery, and people taking blood thinners, such as warfarin (brand name Coumadin®).

Garlic bulbs are sometimes contaminated with the bacterium Clostridium botulinum. C. botulinum can grow and produce botulinum toxin in garlic-in-oil products that are not refrigerated and do not contain antibacterial agents.

In addition, chemical burns, contact dermatitis, and bronchial asthma can occur when garlic is applied to the skin. Garlic should also be avoided by people who are prone to stomach conditions, such as ulcers, as it can exacerbate the condition or cause new ones.

Chapter 9: Red Wine and Cancer Prevention

Red wine is a rich source of biologically active phytochemicals, chemicals found in plants. Particular compounds called polyphenols found in red wine—such as catechins and resveratrol—are thought to have antioxidant or anticancer properties.

What are polyphenols and how do they prevent cancer?

Polyphenols are antioxidant compounds found in the skin and seeds of grapes. When wine is made from these grapes, the alcohol produced by the fermentation process dissolves the polyphenols contained in the skin and seeds. Red wine contains more polyphenols than white wine because the making of white wine requires the removal of the skins after the grapes are crushed. The phenols in red wine include catechin, gallic acid, and epicatechin.

Polyphenols have been found to have antioxidant properties. Antioxidants are substances that protect cells from oxidative damage caused by molecules called free radicals. These chemicals can damage important parts of cells, including proteins, membranes, and DNA. Cellular damage caused by free radicals has been implicated in the development of cancer. Research on the antioxidants found in red wine has shown that they may help inhibit the development of certain cancers.

What is resveratrol and how does it prevent cancer?

Resveratrol is a type of polyphenol called a phytoalexin, a class of compounds produced as part of a plant's defense system against disease. It is produced in the plant in response to an invading fungus, stress, injury, infection, or ultraviolet irradiation. Red wine contains high levels of resveratrol, as do grapes, raspberries, peanuts, and other plants.

Resveratrol has been shown to reduce tumor incidence in animals by affecting one or more stages of cancer development. It has been shown to inhibit growth of many types of cancer cells in culture. Evidence also exists that it can reduce inflammation. It also reduces activation of NF kappa B, a protein produced by the body's immune system when it is under attack. This protein affects cancer cell growth and metastasis. Resveratrol is also an antioxidant.

What have red wine studies found?

The cell and animal studies of red wine have examined effects in several cancers, including leukemia, skin, breast, and prostate cancers. Scientists are studying resveratrol to learn more about its cancer preventive activities. Recent evidence from animal studies suggests this anti-inflammatory compound may be an effective chemopreventive agent in three stages of the cancer process: Initiation, promotion, and progression.

Research studies published in the *International Journal of Cancer* show that drinking a glass of red wine a day may cut a man's risk of prostate cancer in half and that the protective effect appears to be strongest against the most aggressive forms of the disease. It was also seen that men who consumed four or more 4-ounce glasses of red wine per week have a 60 percent lower incidence of the more aggressive types of prostate cancer.

However, studies of the association between red wine consumption and cancer in humans are in their initial stages. Although consumption of large amounts of alcoholic beverages may increase the risk of some cancers, there is growing evidence that the health benefits of red wine are related to its nonalcoholic components.

Chapter 10: Calcium and Cancer Prevention

What is calcium?

Calcium is an essential dietary mineral commonly found in milk, yogurt, cheese, and dark green vegetables. It also is found in certain grains, legumes (including peas, beans, lentils, and peanuts), and nuts.

Calcium is a major component of bones and teeth. It also is required for the clotting of blood to stop bleeding and for normal functioning of the nerves, muscles, and heart.

How much calcium is needed for good health?

Calcium is an important part of a healthy diet; however, the recommended intake differs according to age. As can be seen in the following table, the highest recommended intake is for children and adolescents between the ages of 9 and 18, when bones are growing rapidly.

Dietary Recommendations for Calcium, Males and Females

Age Group	Dietary Recommendations (mg*/day)

0-6 months	210 mg
7-12 months	270 mg
1-3 years	500 mg
4-8 years	800 mg
9-18 years	1300 mg
19-50 years	1000 mg
51 years and older	1200 mg

*mg = milligram

For adults (including women who are pregnant or breastfeeding) and for children age 1 or older, the safe upper limit of calcium intake is 2.5 grams (or 2500 mg) per day. Too much calcium in the diet and from dietary supplements can lead to unwanted side effects.

The U.S. Department of Agriculture's 1994–1996 Continuing Survey of Food Intakes by Individuals showed that the average daily calcium intakes in the United States for males and females over age 9 were 925 mg and 657 mg, respectively, or less than the recommended intake.

How much calcium is in foods and calcium supplements?

Calcium is found in many foods. Foods high in calcium include dairy products, dark green vegetables, some soy products, fish, nuts, and legumes. The following table shows how much calcium is contained in some common foods.

Calcium Amounts in Some Common Foods

Food, Standard Amount	Calcium (mg)
Fruit yogurt, low-fat yogurt, 8 ounces	345
Mozzarella cheese, part-skim, 1.5 ounces	311
Fat-free (skim) milk, 1 cup	306
Sardines, Atlantic, in oil, drained, 3 ounces	325
Tofu, firm, prepared with nigari, ½ cup	253
Spinach, cooked from frozen, ½ cup	146
White beans, canned, ½ cup	96

Packaged foods are required to have a Nutrition Facts label. On foods that contain calcium, this label lists how much calcium there is in each serving of the packaged food. However, the Nutrition Facts labels on packaged foods do not list the calcium content in mg. They only provide the Percent Daily Value (%DV), which is the amount one serving of a food item contributes to the total amount of calcium you need each day. The %DV for calcium is based on a recommended Daily Value of 1000 mg per day. Therefore, a food with 20%DV or more contributes a fair amount of a person's daily total, whereas a food with 5%DV or less contributes only a little. As an example, 1 cup of milk provides 300 mg of calcium and 30%DV.

Calcium supplements most often contain either calcium carbonate or calcium citrate, which are calcium salts. Sometimes, they contain both compounds. Calcium carbonate and calcium citrate have different amounts of elemental calcium, which is the actual amount of usable calcium in a supplement. Specifically, calcium carbonate has about 40 percent elemental calcium, meaning that 500 mg of calcium carbonate actually contains 200 mg of elemental calcium or 20%DV. In contrast, calcium citrate has approximately 21 percent elemental calcium. Therefore, nearly twice as much calcium citrate is needed to obtain the equivalent amount of elemental calcium as in calcium carbonate. Calcium supplements may also contain other calcium salts, but the body may not be able to use the calcium in these compounds. As with food labels, you should look at the Nutrition Facts label on a supplement to determine how much calcium it contains.

Is it safe to take calcium supplements?

For most people, it is safe to eat foods containing calcium and to take calcium supplements that together do not exceed the tolerable upper intake level of 2.5 grams of calcium per day. This upper level for daily calcium intake in adults is the highest level that likely will not pose risks of unwanted side effects in the general population. The upper level of 2.5 grams a day is an average recommendation for all healthy people who are older than a year, regardless of gender. Consuming too much calcium—in excess of 5 grams a day, or 3 grams a day in people with existing kidney problems— can lead to several harmful side effects. Most of these side effects result from people taking too many calcium supplements. Rare harmful side effects from excess calcium include kidney stones, hypercalcemia (too much calcium in the blood), and kidney failure. In addition, excessive consumption of milk (which is high in calcium) and some types of antacids, especially antacids containing calcium carbonate or sodium bicarbonate (baking soda), over a long period of time can cause milk-alkali syndrome, a condition

that can also lead to calcium deposits in the kidneys and
other tissues and to kidney failure.

Is there evidence that calcium may help reduce the risk of colorectal cancer?

The results of epidemiologic studies regarding the
relationship between calcium intake and colorectal cancer
risk have not always been consistent.

In the American Cancer Society's Cancer Prevention Study II
Nutrition Cohort, the diet, medical history, and lifestyle of
more than 120,000 men and women were analyzed. Men and
women who had the highest intakes of calcium through both
their diet and supplement use had a modestly reduced risk of
colorectal cancer compared with those who had the lowest
calcium intakes. However, the benefit from calcium appeared
to plateau, or level off, at an intake of approximately 1200
mg per day. When calcium from the diet was analyzed by
itself, no reduction in colorectal cancer risk was found.
However, the use of calcium supplements in any amount was
associated with reduced risk. This association was strongest
(a 31 percent reduction in risk) for people who took calcium
supplements of 500 mg per day or more.

A stronger relationship between calcium intake and
colorectal cancer risk was found when participants of the

Nurses' Health Study and the Health Professionals Follow-up Study were combined in an analysis that included more than 135,000 men and women. Individuals who had a calcium intake of more than 700 mg per day had a 35 percent to 45 percent reduced risk of cancer of the distal (lower) part of the colon than those who had a calcium intake of 500 mg or less per day. No association was found between calcium intake and risk of cancer of the proximal (middle and upper) part of the colon. Another large study of Finnish men showed a similar relationship between higher calcium intake and reduced risk of colorectal cancer. This study, however, did not evaluate proximal and distal colorectal cancers separately.

In a study that included more than 61,000 Swedish women, colorectal cancer risk was approximately 28 percent lower among individuals who had the highest calcium intakes (approximately 800–1000 mg per day) compared with those with the lowest calcium intakes (approximately 400–500 mg per day). Data from this study also suggested that the benefit associated with calcium was limited to the distal colon. In a study that involved more than 34,000 postmenopausal Iowa women, high intakes of calcium (approximately 1280 mg per day or more) compared with lower calcium intakes (approximately 800 mg per day or less) from both the diet and supplements were associated with a 41 percent reduction in risk of rectal cancer. Reduced risks of rectal cancer were also observed for dietary calcium alone and supplemental calcium alone, but these associations were not statistically significant.

In an analysis involving more than 293,000 men and 198,000 women in the National Institutes of Health-American Association of Retired Persons (NIH-AARP) Diet and Health Study, high intakes of total calcium, dietary calcium, and supplemental calcium were associated with an approximately 20 percent lower risk of colorectal cancer among men and an approximately 30 percent lower risk of colorectal cancer among women.

Findings from two large randomized, placebo-controlled clinical trials, the Calcium Polyp Prevention Study and the European Cancer Prevention Organisation Intervention Study showed that daily supplementation with 1200 to 2000 mg elemental calcium was associated with a reduced risk of recurrence of colorectal polyps known as adenomas in both men and women. Adenomas are thought to be the precursors of most colorectal cancers. In these trials, individuals who previously had one or more large adenomas removed during colonoscopy were randomly assigned to receive calcium supplementation or a placebo, and the rates of polyp recurrence and other factors were compared between the groups.

The Calcium Polyp Prevention Study involved 930 participants who were randomly assigned to receive 3 grams of calcium carbonate (1200 mg elemental calcium) daily for 4 years or a placebo and then receive follow-up colonoscopies approximately 9 months later and again 3 years after that. Compared with those in the placebo group, the individuals assigned to take calcium had about a 20 percent lower risk of adenoma recurrence.

The European Cancer Prevention Organisation Intervention Study involved 665 participants who were randomly assigned to one of three treatment groups: 2 grams of elemental calcium daily (from calcium gluconolactate and calcium carbonate), 3 grams of fiber supplementation daily, or a placebo. The results showed that calcium supplementation was associated with a modest reduction in the risk of adenoma recurrence, but this finding was not statistically significant.

The results of another clinical trial conducted as part of the Women's Health Initiative showed that supplementation with 1000 mg elemental calcium (from calcium carbonate) per day for an average duration of 7 years was not associated with a reduced risk of colorectal cancer. The calcium supplements in this trial also contained vitamin D (400 international units [IU]). During the trial, 128 cases of invasive colorectal cancer were diagnosed in the supplementation group and 126 cases were diagnosed in the placebo group.

In 2007, the World Cancer Research Fund/American Institute for Cancer Research (WCRF/AICR) published the most authoritative review of existing evidence relating food, nutrition, and physical activity to cancer risk. The report concluded that calcium probably has a protective effect against colorectal cancer.

Is there evidence that calcium can help reduce the risk of other cancers?

The results of some studies suggest that a high calcium intake may decrease the risk of one or more types of cancer, whereas other studies suggest that a high calcium intake may actually increase the risk of prostate cancer.

In a randomized trial that included nearly 1,200 healthy, postmenopausal Nebraska women, individuals were randomly assigned to receive daily calcium supplementation alone (300–600 mg elemental calcium), calcium supplementation (300–600 mg elemental calcium) combined with vitamin D supplementation (1000 IU), or a placebo for 4 years. The incidence of all cancers combined was approximately 60 percent lower for women who took the calcium plus vitamin D supplements compared with women who took the placebo. A lower risk of all cancers combined was also observed for women who took calcium supplements alone, but this finding was not statistically significant. The numbers of individual types of cancer diagnosed during this study were too low to be able to draw reliable conclusions about cancer-specific protective effects.

The results of some but not all studies suggest that a high intake of calcium may increase the risk of prostate cancer. For example, the European Prospective Investigation into Cancer and Nutrition analyzed the intakes of animal foods (meat, poultry, fish, dairy products, etc.), protein, and calcium in relation to prostate cancer risk among more than 142,000 men and found that a high intake of protein or calcium from dairy products was associated with an increased risk of prostate cancer. Calcium from nondairy sources, however, was not associated with increased risk. In addition, a prospective analysis of dairy product and calcium intakes among more than 29,000 men participating in the National Cancer Institute's (NCI) Prostate, Lung, Colorectal, and Ovarian (PLCO) Cancer Screening Trial showed increased risks for prostate cancer associated with high dietary intakes of calcium and dairy products, particularly low-fat dairy products. Calcium from supplements was not associated with increased prostate cancer risk. In contrast, results from the NIH-AARP Diet and Health Study showed no increased risk of prostate cancer associated with total calcium, dietary calcium, or supplemental calcium intakes. Other studies have suggested that intakes of low-fat milk, lactose, and calcium from dairy products may reduce the risk of ovarian cancer, but this risk reduction has not been found in all studies.

An analysis from the Nurses' Health Study that included more than 3,000 women found that higher calcium intakes (more than 800 mg per day) from dairy products— particularly low-fat or nonfat milk, yogurt, and cheese— compared with lower calcium intakes (200 mg or less per day) from dairy products was associated with a reduced risk of breast cancer among premenopausal but not postmenopausal women. Calcium from nondairy sources was not associated with a reduction in risk. Another analysis that involved more than 30,000 women in the Women's Health Study found a reduced risk of breast cancer associated with higher (1366 mg per day or more) versus lower (less than 617 mg per day) total intakes of calcium among premenopausal but not postmenopausal women. In this study, higher versus lower calcium intakes from the diet, from supplements, and from total dairy products were not associated with reduced risk.

How might calcium help prevent cancer?

Although the exact mechanism by which calcium may help reduce the risk of colorectal cancer is unclear, researchers know that, at the biochemical level, calcium binds to bile acids and fatty acids in the gastrointestinal tract to form insoluble complexes known as calcium soaps. This reduces the ability of the acids (or their metabolites) to damage cells in the lining of the colon and stimulate cell proliferation to repair the damage. Calcium may also act directly to reduce cell proliferation in the lining of the colon or cause proliferating colon cells to undergo differentiation, which, in turn, leads to a reduction in cell proliferation. Calcium also may improve signaling within cells and cause cancer cells to differentiate and/or die.

How does the body absorb calcium from foods and supplements?

Calcium is absorbed passively (no cellular energy required) in the intestines by diffusing through the spaces between cells. It is also absorbed actively (cellular energy required) through intestinal cells by binding to a transport protein known as calbindin. The production of calbindin is dependent on vitamin D.

Chapter 11: Statins and Cancer Prevention

What are statins?

Statins are a type of drug taken by millions of Americans to lower cholesterol. This class of drugs works by blocking an enzyme known as HMG-CoA (3-hydroxy-3-methyglutaryl COA) reductase, which the body needs to make cholesterol. Statins help to treat and prevent heart disease by lowering blood cholesterol. In the United States, statins available by prescription include atorvastatin (Lipitor™), lovastatin (Mevacor™), pravastatin (Pravachol™), and simvastatin (Zocor™). In the United States, statins are available by prescription only.

Can statins prevent cancer?

Animal research and ongoing observation of people who take statins suggest that these drugs may lower the risk of certain cancers, including colorectal and skin cancers. Statins' known benefits in preventing cardiovascular disease, along with years of strong evidence that these agents are relatively safe, have led researchers to explore whether statins have the potential to prevent cancer. People should not take statins for cancer prevention outside of a clinical trial.

Why do scientists think statins might prevent cancer?

By exploring the effects of statins on the process of cancer at the molecular level, researchers have found that statins work against critical cellular functions that may help control tumor initiation, tumor growth, and metastasis. Specifically, statins reduce (or block) the activity of the enzyme HMG-CoA reductase and thereby reduce the levels of mevalonate and its associated products. The mevalonate pathway plays a role in cell membrane integrity, cell signaling, protein synthesis, and cell cycle progression, all of which are potential areas of intervention to arrest the cancer process.

What are the common side effects of statins?

Although generally well-tolerated, statins have been associated with muscle pain (myopathy) and liver toxicity (hepatotoxicity). People who take statins should be monitored by their health care providers for these reasons.

What evidence is there that statins may have an effect on colorectal cancer?

Studies have shown that statins inhibit the growth of colon cancer cells grown in the laboratory. Consistent preventive effects of certain statins against colon cancer were first described in cancer studies in rodents published in 1994. Some human observational studies have since suggested that statins may have protective effects against colorectal cancer. Most recently, researchers from the University of Michigan, collaborating with researchers in Israel, compared the use of statins among 1,953 patients who were diagnosed with colorectal cancer and 2,015 other people who did not have the disease. This study specifically associated a 47 percent reduction in the risk of colorectal cancer with statin use (as opposed to the use of another type of lipid-lowering drug, fibrates). [Statins and the risk of colorectal cancer. Poynter, JN., et al. *New England Journal of Medicine*, May 26, 2005, (352:2184–92].

What evidence is there that lipid-lowering drugs can prevent skin cancer?

Two large cardiovascular clinical trials have demonstrated a significant reduction in skin cancer among patients taking lipid-lowering drugs. Although clinical data do not consistently show a decreased risk of skin cancer with statin use, various human trials and preclinical studies suggest that statins may have chemopreventive activity against skin cancer.

Chapter 12: Vitamin D and Cancer Prevention

- Vitamin D is essential for the formation, growth, and repair of bones and for normal calcium absorption and immune function. It is obtained primarily through exposure of the skin to ultraviolet radiation in sunlight, but it can also be obtained from some foods and dietary supplements.

- Some studies suggest that higher intakes of vitamin D from food and/or supplements and higher levels of vitamin D in the blood are associated with reduced risks of colorectal cancer; however, the research results overall have been inconsistent.

- Whether vitamin D is associated with reduced risks of other cancers, including breast, prostate, and pancreatic cancers, remains unclear.

- The National Cancer Institute (NCI) does not recommend for or against the use of vitamin D supplements to reduce the risk of colorectal or any other type of cancer.

- Note: The information in this fact sheet is not to be used as the basis for making health claims about products containing vitamin D.

What is vitamin D?

Vitamin D is technically not a vitamin. It is the name given to a group of fat-soluble prohormones (substances that are precursors to hormones that usually have little hormonal activity by themselves). Two major forms of vitamin D that are important to humans are vitamin D2, or ergocalciferol, and vitamin D3, or cholecalciferol. Vitamin D2 is made naturally by plants, and vitamin D3 is made naturally by the body when the skin is exposed to ultraviolet radiation (in particular, UVB radiation) in sunlight. Vitamin D2 and vitamin D3 can also be commercially manufactured.

The active form of vitamin D in the body is 1,25-dihydroxyvitamin D, or calcitriol, which can be made from either vitamin D2 or vitamin D3. To make the active form, vitamin D2 and vitamin D3 are modified in the liver to produce 25-hydroxyvitamin D, which travels through the blood to the kidneys, where it is modified further to make 1,25-dihydroxyvitamin D.

Vitamin D is involved in a number of processes that are essential for good health, including the following:

- It helps improve muscle strength and immune function.
- It helps reduce inflammation.
- It promotes the absorption of calcium from the small intestine.
- It helps maintain adequate blood levels of the calcium and phosphate needed for bone formation, mineralization (incorporating minerals to increase strength and density), growth, and repair.

Most people get the vitamin D they need through sunlight exposure. It can also be obtained through the diet, but very few foods naturally contain vitamin D. These foods include fatty fish, fish liver oil, and eggs. Smaller amounts are found in meat and cheese. Most dietary vitamin D comes from fortified foods, such as milk, juices, yogurt, bread, and breakfast cereals. Vitamin D can also be obtained through dietary supplements. Fortified foods and dietary supplements usually contain either vitamin D2 or vitamin D3. A person's vitamin D status is usually checked by measuring the level of 25-hydroxyvitamin D in their blood serum.

How much vitamin D is needed for health?

A serum level of 25-hydroxyvitamin D lower than 15 nanograms per milliliter (ng/mL)—equivalent to 37.5 nanomoles per liter (nmol/L)—is generally considered inadequate for a healthy person to maintain bone health and normal calcium metabolism. However, some experts say that this may be on the low side, and the 2005 Dietary Guidelines for Americans notes that the optimal level may be as high as 80 nmol/L. A serum level below 11 ng/mL (27.5 nmol/L) is consistent with vitamin D deficiency in infants, neonates, and young children. The Institute of Medicine of the National Academies has developed the following recommended daily intakes of vitamin D (on the assumption that vitamin D3 is not being made in the skin through sun exposure).

Age	Recommended Minimum Vitamin D Intake (μg/day and IU/day)
Birth to 50 years	5 μg (=200 IU)
51-70 years	10 μg (=400 IU)
71+ years	15 μg (=600 IU)
Pregnancy	5 μg (=200 IU)
Lactation	5 μg (=200 IU)

μg = microgram; 1 μg = 40 International Units (IU)

The 2005 *Dietary Guidelines for Americans* recommends that older adults, people with dark skin, and people exposed to insufficient sunlight should consume extra vitamin D from vitamin D-fortified foods and/or supplements.

People are more likely to not get enough vitamin D than to get too much. However, excessive intake of any nutrient, including vitamin D, can cause toxic effects (see Question 5). Excessive sun exposure does not cause vitamin D toxicity.

How much vitamin D is in fortified foods and supplements?

Fortification of foods with vitamin D in the United States is carefully regulated. Vitamin D fortification is allowed for milk and milk products, cereal flours and related products, margarine, soy-based food products, and fruit juices and fruit juice drinks. Milk is usually fortified with 2.5 μg (100 IU) vitamin D per cup. Some yogurts are now fortified with vitamin D. Cheese, ice cream, and other dairy products made from milk are generally not fortified with vitamin D. To see if a food product has been fortified, check the food label. The amount of vitamin D in multivitamins and other dietary supplements typically ranges from 10 μg (400 IU) to 50 μg (2,000 IU).

Is it safe to take vitamin D supplements?

Vitamin D toxicity is more likely to occur from high intakes of dietary supplements than from high intakes of vitamin D-fortified foods. For most children and adults, the tolerable upper intake level (UL) of vitamin D intake from foods and supplements is 25 μg (1,000 IU) per day for those less than 1 year of age and 50 μg (2,000 IU) per day for older individuals. The UL is the highest level of daily intake (from all sources combined) that is likely to pose no risk of adverse effects for almost all people.

Excessive vitamin D intake is toxic because it increases calcium levels. Increased calcium levels can lead to calcinosis (the deposit of calcium salts in soft tissues of the body, such as the kidneys, heart, and lungs) and hypercalcemia (high blood levels of calcium). Symptoms of excessive vitamin D intake may include heart rhythm abnormalities; mental status changes, such as confusion; pain; conjunctivitis; anorexia; fever; chills; thirst; vomiting; and weight loss.

Is there a role for vitamin D in reducing cancer risk?

A large number of scientific studies have investigated a possible role for vitamin D in cancer prevention.

- The first results came from epidemiologic studies known as geographic correlation studies. In these studies, an inverse relationship was found between sunlight exposure levels in a given geographic area and the rates of incidence and death for certain cancers in that area. Individuals living in southern latitudes were found to have lower rates of incidence and death for these cancers than those living at northern latitudes. Because sunlight/UV exposure is necessary for the production of vitamin D3, researchers hypothesized that variation in vitamin D levels accounted for the observed relationships.

- Evidence of a possible cancer-protective role for vitamin D has also been found in laboratory studies of the effect of vitamin D treatment on cancer cells in culture. In these studies, vitamin D promoted the differentiation and death (apoptosis) of cancer cells, and it slowed their proliferation.

- Randomized clinical trials designed to investigate the effects of vitamin D intake on bone health have suggested that higher vitamin D intakes may reduce the risk of cancer. One study involved nearly 1,200 healthy postmenopausal women who took daily supplements of calcium (1,400 mg or 1,500 mg) and vitamin D (25 µg vitamin D, or 1,100 IU—a relatively large dose) or a placebo for 4 years. The women who took the supplements had a 60 percent lower overall incidence of cancer; however, the study did not include a vitamin D-only group. Moreover, the primary outcome of the study was fracture incidence; it was not designed to measure cancer incidence. This limits the ability to draw conclusions about the effect of vitamin D intake on cancer risk.

- A number of observational studies have investigated whether people with higher vitamin D levels or intake have lower risks of specific cancers, particularly colorectal cancer and breast cancer. Associations of vitamin D with risks of prostate, pancreatic, and other, rarer cancers have also been examined. These studies have yielded inconsistent results, most likely because of the challenges of conducting observational studies of diet. Information about dietary intakes is obtained from the participants through the use of food frequency questionnaires, diet records, or interviews in which the participants are asked to recall information about their dietary intakes. Information collected in this manner can be inaccurate. In addition, only recently has a comprehensive food composition database with vitamin D values for the U.S. food supply become available. Other dietary components or energy balance may also modify vitamin D metabolism.

- Measuring blood levels of 25-hydroxyvitamin D to determine vitamin D status avoids some of the limitations of assessing dietary intake. However, vitamin D levels in the blood vary by race, with the season, and possibly with the activity of genes whose products are involved in vitamin D transport and metabolism. These variations complicate the interpretation of studies that measure the concentration of vitamin D in serum at a single point in time.

- Finally, it is difficult to separate the effects of vitamin D and calcium because of the complicated biological interactions between these substances. To fully understand the effect of vitamin D on cancer and other health outcomes, new randomized trials will need to be carried out.

However, the appropriate dose of vitamin D to use in such trials is still not clear

Is there evidence that vitamin D can help reduce the risk of colorectal cancer?

Epidemiologic studies of the association between vitamin D and the risk of colorectal cancer have provided some indications that higher levels of intake are associated with a reduced risk. However, the data are inconsistent.

In the American Cancer Society's Cancer Prevention Study (CPS) II Nutrition Cohort, the diet, medical history, and lifestyle of more than 120,000 men and women were analyzed. Men who had the highest intakes of vitamin D through both their diet and supplement use (greater than 13 µg, or 525 IU, per day) had a slightly lower risk of colorectal cancer than men who had the lowest vitamin D intakes. However, this association was not observed among women. In a pooled analysis of data from 10 cohort studies (including the CPS II cohort), individuals with the highest dietary vitamin D intakes had a slightly lower risk of colorectal cancer than those with the lowest intakes, but the reduction in risk was not statistically significant.

In the Women's Health Initiative randomized trial, healthy postmenopausal women took daily supplements that contained both calcium (1,000 mg) and vitamin D (10 μg, or 400 IU) or a placebo for an average of 7 years. Supplementation did not reduce the incidence of colorectal cancer. However, some scientists have raised the possibility that the relatively low level of vitamin D supplementation and the short duration of participant follow-up might account for the negative results.

At least one epidemiologic study has reported an association between vitamin D and reduced mortality from colorectal cancer. Among the 16,818 participants in the Third National Health and Nutrition Examination Survey, those with higher vitamin D blood levels ($\geq$80 nmol/L) had a 72 percent lower risk of colorectal cancer death than those with lower vitamin D blood levels (< 50 nmol/L).

Most colorectal cancers develop from pre-existing colorectal adenomas, and interventions that reduce the risk of adenoma development or recurrence are likely to reduce the risk of colorectal cancer. Several large studies have investigated the association of vitamin D intake or serum status with adenoma risk.

A cohort from the National Cancer Institute (NCI)-sponsored Polyp Prevention Trial (PPT) was evaluated for the association of vitamin D intake with recurrence of colorectal adenomas in individuals who previously had one or more adenomas removed during a qualifying colonoscopy. PPT was a multicenter randomized clinical trial to determine the effects of a diet high in fiber, fruits, and vegetables and low in fat on adenoma recurrence. The detailed dietary information obtained during the trial allowed the researchers to investigate the association between additional dietary factors and adenoma recurrence. Total vitamin D intake (that is, from dietary sources and supplements combined) was not associated with a reduced risk of adenoma recurrence. However, individuals who used any amount of vitamin D supplements had a lower risk of adenoma recurrence.

In another study, the vitamin D intakes of 3,000 people from several Veterans Affairs medical centers were examined to determine whether there was an association between intake and advanced colorectal neoplasia (an outcome that included high-risk adenomas as well as colon cancer). Individuals with the highest vitamin D intakes (more than 16 μg, or 645 IU, per day) had a lower risk of developing advanced neoplasia than those with lower intakes.

A pooled analysis of data from these and a number of other observational studies found that higher circulating levels of vitamin D and higher vitamin D intakes were associated with lower risks of colorectal adenoma. Inverse associations were seen with both dietary and total vitamin D intake but not with supplemental vitamin D intake. However, the associations with dietary intake were not statistically significant.

Another large, NCI-sponsored randomized, placebo-controlled trial explored the effects of calcium supplementation and blood levels of vitamin D on adenoma recurrence. Calcium supplementation reduced the risk of adenoma recurrence only in individuals with vitamin D blood levels above 73 nmol/L. Among individuals with vitamin D levels at or below this level, calcium supplementation was not associated with a reduced risk.

Is there evidence that vitamin D can help reduce breast cancer risk?

Epidemiologic studies of the association between vitamin D and breast cancer risk have had conflicting results. Although several studies have suggested an inverse association between vitamin D intake and the risk of breast cancer, others have shown no association or even a positive association (that is, individuals with higher intakes had higher risks). A meta-analysis of six studies that investigated the relationship between vitamin D intake and breast cancer risk found no association. However, most women in these studies had relatively low vitamin D intakes, and, when the analysis was restricted to women with the highest vitamin D intakes (>10 μg, or 400 IU, per day), their breast cancer risks were lower than those of women with the lowest intakes (typically <1.25 μg, or 50 IU, per day).

In the Women's Health Initiative, calcium plus vitamin D supplementation for an average of 7 years did not reduce the incidence of invasive breast cancer compared with placebo. The association between blood levels of vitamin D and breast cancer risk was examined in a cohort of postmenopausal women who were enrolled in NCI's Prostate, Lung, Colorectal, and Ovarian (PLCO) Cancer Screening Trial and from whom blood was drawn at study entry. During the subsequent follow-up period, 1,005 of these women developed breast cancer. When researchers compared the blood vitamin D levels of these women with those of 1,005 similar control women who did not develop breast cancer, they found no association between vitamin D status and risk of breast cancer.

Is there evidence that vitamin D can help reduce prostate cancer risk?

Some geographic correlation studies have suggested that men exposed to higher levels of sunlight may have a lower risk of prostate cancer. Although some epidemiologic studies have suggested that men with higher vitamin D levels have an increased risk of prostate cancer, most studies have not shown such an association.

In one relatively large study of men diagnosed 1 to 8 years after their blood was drawn, higher vitamin D blood levels were not associated with a lower risk of prostate cancer overall. Indeed, there was some evidence that men with higher vitamin D levels had an increased risk for aggressive disease.

In another study, the European Prospective Investigation into Cancer and Nutrition (EPIC), blood samples obtained at study entry were examined for 652 men who developed prostate cancer during follow-up and 752 matched control subjects. No association was observed between serum vitamin D levels and risk of prostate cancer, either overall or by cancer stage.

Is there evidence that vitamin D can help reduce pancreatic cancer risk?

There is conflicting evidence about vitamin D's relationship to risk of pancreatic cancer. A study of more than 120,000 men and women from the Health Professionals Follow-Up Study and the Nurses' Health Study showed that participants with higher dietary intake of vitamin D had progressively lower risk of pancreatic cancer, compared with those who had the lowest intake. The estimates of vitamin D intake were based on detailed dietary information provided through questionnaires. Participants were followed for 16 years for the incidence of pancreatic cancer, and 365 cases were identified.

In a study of men and women enrolled in the PLCO Screening Trial, no association between vitamin D level and pancreatic cancer risk was observed. The PLCO study examined vitamin D levels in blood from 184 individuals who were diagnosed with pancreatic cancer during nearly 12 years of follow-up and 368 matched cancer-free control subjects. In contrast, among Finnish male smokers participating in the Alpha-Tocopherol, Beta-Carotene (ATBC) Cancer Prevention Study, higher blood levels of vitamin D were associated with an increased risk of pancreatic cancer. More recently, in the NCI Cohort Consortium Vitamin D Pooling Project of Rarer Cancers, men and women with the highest blood vitamin D levels (greater than 100 nmol/L, or 40 ng/mL) had twice the pancreatic cancer risk of men and women whose blood vitamin D levels were in the normal range of 50-75 nmol/L (20-30 ng/mL).

Is there evidence that vitamin D can help reduce the risk of other rare cancers?

A recent large collaborative effort analyzed data from 10 prospective cohort studies to examine whether vitamin D levels in blood were associated with seven rare cancers. The NCI Cohort Consortium Vitamin D Pooling Project of Rarer Cancers included information on blood vitamin D levels and incidence of rare cancers in a subset of more than 12,000 men and women. The researchers matched participants on date and season of blood draw and used other statistical techniques to adjust for seasonal variation in blood vitamin D levels. When the data from the different studies were pooled, there was no overall association between vitamin D level and risk of non-Hodgkin lymphoma or cancers of the endometrium, esophagus, stomach, kidney, or ovary. An increased risk of pancreatic cancer was observed in those with the highest blood levels of vitamin D (greater than 100 nmol/L or 40 ng/mL).

What are the possible mechanisms by which vitamin D may modify cancer risk?

Mechanisms by which vitamin D may modify cancer risk are not fully understood. Laboratory studies have shown that vitamin D promotes cellular differentiation, decreases cancer cell growth, and stimulates apoptosis.

Vitamin D acts on cells by binding to the vitamin D receptor (VDR). The VDR is a regulator of gene transcription that is found in the nucleus of cells. Vitamin D-bound VDR binds to the retinoid-X receptor (RXR), and the resulting complex activates the expression of specific genes. Among the many genes regulated by vitamin D are those that produce the proteins calbindin and TPRV6, both of which are involved in the absorption of calcium by intestinal cells. Another vitamin D-regulated gene is CYP3A4, whose protein product detoxifies the bile acid lithocholic acid (LCA). LCA is believed to damage the DNA of intestinal cells and may promote colon carcinogenesis. Stimulating the production of a detoxifying enzyme by vitamin D could explain a protective role for vitamin D against colon cancer.

Further insight into the mechanisms by which vitamin D might modify cancer risk could come from study of the vitamin D receptor itself. A large number of variant forms of the VDR gene have been identified, some of which are known to alter the structure or function of the VDR protein. Some of these variants have been linked to risk for certain cancers, including prostate, colorectal, breast, bladder, and melanoma. The association of VDR variants with cancer risk differs by cancer site and appears to be modified by environmental exposures, such as diet and sun exposure.

How can people get enough sunlight for vitamin D synthesis while minimizing the risk of skin cancer?

Although people obtain some vitamin D from dietary sources, most vitamin D is made in the body after the skin is exposed to sunlight. Despite the known and potential health benefits of vitamin D, increasing sun exposure increases the risk of skin cancer. In general, most experts believe that people should continue to use sun protection when UV levels are moderate or higher. Some researchers have suggested that brief daily exposure to UV will ensure adequate vitamin D production, but many variables (such as skin color, latitude, and season) can affect the production of vitamin D, and such recommendations have proven controversial. Other experts recommend vitamin D supplementation to avoid the problem of increasing skin cancer risk.

Physical Activity and Cancer

What is physical activity?

Physical activity is any bodily movement produced by skeletal muscles; such movement results in an expenditure of energy. Physical activity is a critical component of energy balance, a term used to describe how weight, diet, and physical activity influence health, including cancer risk.

How is physical activity related to health?

Researchers have established that regular physical activity can improve health by:

Helping to control weight.

- Maintaining healthy bones, muscles, and joints.
- Reducing the risk of developing high blood pressure and diabetes.
- Promoting psychological well-being.
- Reducing the risk of death from heart disease.
- Reducing the risk of premature death.

In addition to these health benefits, researchers are learning that physical activity can also affect the risk of cancer. There is convincing evidence that physical activity is associated with a reduced risk of cancers of the colon and breast. Several studies also have reported links between physical activity and a reduced risk of cancers of the prostate, lung, and lining of the uterus (endometrial cancer). Despite these health benefits, recent studies have shown that more than 50 percent of Americans do not engage in enough regular physical activity.

How much physical activity do adults need?

The Centers for Disease Control and Prevention (CDC) recommend that adults "engage in moderate-intensity physical activity for at least 30 minutes on five or more days of the week," or "engage in vigorous-intensity physical activity for at least 20 minutes on three or more days of the week".

What is the relationship between physical activity and colon cancer risk?

Colorectal cancer has been one of the most extensively studied cancers in relation to physical activity, with more than 50 studies examining this association. Many studies in the United States and around the world have consistently found that adults who increase their physical activity, either in intensity, duration, or frequency, can reduce their risk of developing colon cancer by 30 to 40 percent relative to those who are sedentary regardless of body mass index (BMI), with the greatest risk reduction seen among those who are most active. The magnitude of the protective effect appears greatest with high-intensity activity, although the optimal levels and duration of exercise are still difficult to determine due to differences between studies, making comparisons difficult. It is estimated that 30 to 60 minutes of moderate to vigorous physical activity per day is needed to protect against colon cancer. It is not yet clear at this time whether physical activity has a protective effect for rectal cancer, adenomas, or polyp recurrence.

Physical activity most likely influences the development of colon cancer in multiple ways. Physical activity may protect against colon cancer and tumor development through its role in energy balance, hormone metabolism, insulin regulation, and by decreasing the time the colon is exposed to potential carcinogens. Physical activity has also been found to alter a number of inflammatory and immune factors, some of which may influence colon cancer risk.

What is the relationship between physical activity and breast cancer risk?

The relationship between physical activity and breast cancer incidence has been extensively studied, with over 60 studies published in North America, Europe, Asia, and Australia.

Most studies indicate that physically active women have a lower risk of developing breast cancer than inactive women; however, the amount of risk reduction achieved through physical activity varies widely (between 20 to 80 percent). Although most evidence suggests that physical activity reduces breast cancer risk in both premenopausal and postmenopausal women, high levels of moderate and vigorous physical activity during adolescence may be especially protective. Although a lifetime of regular, vigorous activity is thought to be of greatest benefit, women who increase their physical activity after menopause may also experience a reduced risk compared with inactive women. A number of studies also suggest that the effect of physical activity may be different across levels of BMI, with the greatest benefit seen in women in the normal weight range (generally a BMI under 25 kg/m-squared) in some studies. Existing evidence shows a decreasing risk of breast cancer as the frequency and duration of physical activity increase. Most studies suggest that 30 to 60 minutes per day of moderate- to high-intensity physical activity is associated with a reduction in breast cancer risk.

Researchers have proposed several biological mechanisms to explain the relationship between physical activity and breast cancer development. Physical activity may prevent tumor development by lowering hormone levels, particularly in premenopausal women; lowering levels of insulin and insulin-like growth factor I (IGF-I), improving the immune response; and assisting with weight maintenance to avoid a high body mass and excess body fat.

What is the relationship between physical activity and risk of endometrial cancer?

About 20 studies have examined the role of physical activity on endometrial cancer risk. The results suggest an inverse relationship between physical activity and endometrial cancer incidence. These studies suggest that women who are physically active have a 20 percent to 40 percent reduced risk of endometrial cancer, with the greatest reduction in risk among those with the highest levels of physical activity. Risk does not appear to vary by age.

Changes in body mass and changes in the levels and metabolism of sex hormones, such as estrogen, are the major biological mechanisms thought to explain the association between physical activity and endometrial cancer. However, fewer than half of the studies in this area have also adjusted for the potential effect of postmenopausal hormone use, which may increase the risk of endometrial cancer. A few studies have examined whether the effect of physical activity varies according to the weight of the woman, but the results have been inconsistent.

What is the relationship between physical activity and lung cancer risk?

At least 21 studies have examined the impact of physical activity on the risk of lung cancer. Overall, these studies suggest an inverse association between physical activity and lung cancer risk, with the most physically active individuals experiencing about a 20 percent reduction in risk. An analysis of many existing studies found evidence that higher levels of physical activity protect against lung cancer, but was unable to fully control for the effects of smoking or respiratory disease in estimating the magnitude of the potential benefit. The relationship between physical activity and lung cancer risk is less clear for women than it is for men.

What is the relationship between physical activity and risk of prostate cancer?

Research findings are less consistent about the effect of physical activity on prostate cancer, with at least 36 studies in North America, Europe, and Asia. Overall, the epidemiologic research does not indicate that there is an inverse relationship between physical activity and prostate cancer. Although it is possible that men who are physically active experience a reduction in risk of prostate cancer, the potential biological mechanisms that may explain this association are unknown, but may be related to changes in hormones, energy balance, insulin-like growth factors, immunity, and antioxidant defense mechanisms. One recent study suggested that regular vigorous activity could slow the progression of prostate cancer in men age 65 or older.

How might physical activity affect cancer survivorship?

Research indicates that physical activity after a diagnosis of breast cancer may be beneficial in improving quality of life, reducing fatigue, and assisting with energy balance. Both reduced physical activity and the side effects of treatment have been linked to weight gain after a breast cancer diagnosis. One study found that women who exercised moderately (the equivalent of walking 3 to 5 hours per week at an average pace) after a diagnosis of breast cancer had improved survival rates compared with more sedentary women. The benefit was particularly pronounced in women with hormone responsive tumors. Another study found that a home-based physical activity program had a beneficial effect on the fitness and psychological well-being of previously sedentary women who had completed treatment for early-stage through stage II breast cancer. Increasing physical activity may influence insulin and leptin levels and influence breast cancer prognosis. Although there are several promising studies, it is too early to draw any strong conclusions regarding physical activity and breast cancer survival.

Two additional studies have suggested a protective association of physical activity after colon cancer diagnosis and survival. Researchers examined the relationship between levels of physical activity both before and after a diagnosis of colon cancer in two different observational studies. Whereas levels of pre-diagnosis physical activity were not related to survival, participants with higher levels of physical activity post-diagnosis were less likely to have a cancer recurrence and had increased survival. Although these studies suggest protective effects of physical activity, more research is needed to understand what levels of physical activity provide these benefits.

Other MedicalCenter.com Publications

The Key Facts on Arthritis

The Key Facts on Breast Cancer

The Key Facts on Medicare

The Key Facts on Alzheimer's Disease

The Key Facts on Caring For Someone With

Alzheimer's Disease

The Key Facts on Cancer Series

**All Titles Can Be Found at**

**www.Amazon.com**

www.MedicalCenter.com

www.ingramcontent.com/pod-product-compliance
Lightning Source LLC
Chambersburg PA
CBHW070702290526
45790CB00001B/415